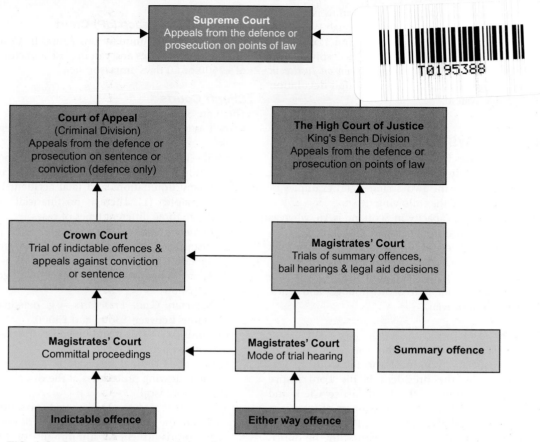

FIG. 1.3 Criminal procedures and appeals.

b. *Second tier courts*—These have either KBD or circuit judges and they try Class 2 offences such as rape and manslaughter.
c. *Third tier courts*—These have either circuit judges or recorders and try Class 3 offences such as grievous bodily harm (GBH) or fraud (Fig. 1.3).

Appeals
- A person convicted by a magistrates' court can appeal to a Crown Court against:
  1. the sentence if the plea was 'guilty'
  2. the sentence or conviction if the plea was 'not guilty'.
- Appeals against Crown Court convictions are heard by the Criminal Division of the Court of Appeal:
  1. from the defendant on the length of sentence and on questions of fact and law
  2. from the prosecution on points of law where the accused has been acquitted.

- There is also a civil division of the Court of Appeal, which hears appeals from certain tribunals and the county and High Courts.
- The final appeal court for both civil and criminal cases is the Supreme Court, but this only hears appeals on points of law and then only in cases where there is public interest in the outcome.
- If there is an issue concerning the interpretation of community law, then the case must be referred to the European Court of Human Rights for a ruling.

Welsh Law
In 2006 the National Assembly for Wales was reformed and renamed as the Senedd by the *Government of Wales Act 2006* and since 2007 they have been able to make primary legislation for Wales. The Senedd generate both primary (known as *Act of Senedd Cymru*) and secondary legislation, but there is no criminal law and it has no impact on English

common law unless the Welsh legislation is a superior form of law. This means that although Welsh law is acknowledged as separate in operation, it is not yet recognised as a separate legal system despite publication of the report of the *'Commission on Justice in Wales'* in 2019, which recommended full devolution of the justice system.

THE LEGAL SYSTEM OF SCOTLAND

English law derives from the Norman Conquest, which Scotland effectively avoided so there are significant variations between the two systems and examples of such differences are the following:

- The age of legal capacity in Scotland is 16, whereas it is 18 in the rest of the United Kingdom.
- Scottish juries consist of 15 jurors and they only ever need to reach a majority verdict.
- In addition to 'guilty' and 'not guilty', there is a third verdict available to Scottish judges and juries, which is 'not proven'.

Judiciary

The highest courts in Scotland comprise the High Court of Justiciary (criminal) and the Court of Session (civil) and the president is the Lord Justice General. His deputy is the Lord Justice Clerk and then there are 35 Lords Commissioners of Justiciary. Criminal law is administered by a Public Prosecutor known as the Lord Advocate, who with the Solicitor General and 12 Advocates-Depute (known collectively as the Crown Counsel) prosecutes cases on behalf of the Crown. The Crown Office is equivalent to the Lord Chief Justice's department but also has a function like that of the CPS. Both examine the evidence in serious criminal cases, decide whether the case should go to trial and the level of court in which it should be held.

Scotland is divided into six regions called Sheriffdoms and each has a Sheriff Principal. He is responsible for the conduct of the courts and for hearing appeals on civil matters. The public prosecutor in the Sheriff and District courts is known as the Procurator Fiscal, who also has a parallel role to the English Coroner. He is a legally qualified member of the civil service whose role is to assess the evidence in each case and decide whether to proceed with the case. The Fiscal acts as the prosecutor in summary cases but in the High Court, his role is as solicitor to the Crown Counsel.

Courts
Justice of the Peace (JP) Court

Operating under summary procedure, JP Courts hear minor criminal cases and can impose a maximum fine of £2500 or 60 days' imprisonment.

Sheriff Courts

There are 39 Sheriff Courts and the presiding judge is known as a Sheriff. There are three main categories of work:

- **Civil**—The Sheriff Courts deal with most civil litigation including adoption, uncontested divorces, company liquidations and fatal accident inquiries (see Chapter 11). There is no financial limit and there are three different types of cases:
  1. *Ordinary Cause Procedures*—e.g. divorce, property disputes, damage claims over £5000 and child welfare
  2. *Simple Cause Procedures*—e.g. debt collection up to £5000
  3. *Summary Cause Procedures*—e.g. personal injury claims between £3000 and £5000.
- **Commissary**—This mainly involves the disposal of a deceased person's estate.
- **Criminal**—Criminal cases are brought under one of the following procedures at the discretion of the Procurator Fiscal:
  1. *Solemn Procedure*—This is used for serious cases where the penalty involves a fine of over £5000 or imprisonment for a minimum of 3 months. The case is heard before a Sheriff and a jury and the Sheriff can refer the case to the High Court for sentencing, as the maximum penalty that he can impose is 5 years' imprisonment or an unlimited fine.
  2. *Summary Procedure*—This is used for lesser cases and they are heard by the Sheriff alone. The maximum sentence that can be imposed is 12 months' imprisonment or a £10,000 fine (Fig. 1.4).

Court of Session

This is the supreme civil court and it is based in Parliament House in Edinburgh. It is divided into two Houses:

1. *Outer House*—This hears more serious civil disputes in the first instance, e.g. medical negligence cases. All cases are prepared and decided by judges called Lords Ordinary. They sit alone or with a jury, but they are subject to review by three or more other judges from the nine judges who form the Inner House.

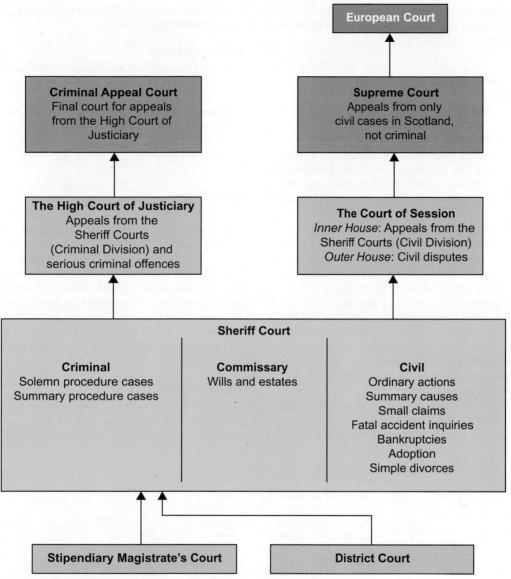

FIG. 1.4 A simplified representation of the court system of Scotland.

2. *Inner House*—This reviews decisions made by the Outer House and hears appeals on civil cases from the Sheriff Courts. It has two divisions with the First Division being chaired by the Lord President and the Second by the Lord Justice Clerk. If neither is available, an Extra Division is formed and chaired by the next most senior judge, but all three divisions have the same authority. Usually, cases are heard by three judges but five or more may sit for more serious cases.

The High Court of Justiciary

This is the supreme criminal court and it is also primarily based in Edinburgh. It has the same judges as the Court of Session, but they are called Lord Commissioners of Justiciary and they wear different robes. The High Court cannot appeal to the Supreme Court. More serious criminal cases, e.g. rape and murder, are heard before a judge and jury and, unlike the Court of Session, the High Court also sits in other towns using Circuit judges. Appeals from the Sheriff Courts are always heard in Edinburgh by a bench of three or more judges.

THE LEGAL SYSTEM OF NORTHERN IRELAND

This is very similar to that of England and Wales.

Superior Courts

The practice and procedure of these Courts, known collectively as the Court of Judicature, is essentially the same as their equivalents in England and Wales and they are all under the jurisdiction of the British Parliament.

- **Court of Appeal**—This comprises the Lord Chief Justice and two Lord Justices of Appeal and sits in the Royal Courts of Justice in Belfast. It has the power to review all civil law decisions of the High Court and all criminal law decisions in the Crown Court.
- **High Court**—This comprises the Lord Chief Justice and five other judges and again sits in Belfast. It has a KBD, which deals with most civil law matters, a Family Division and a Chancery Division for trusts, estates, wills and land matters. It hears more serious criminal and civil cases and appeals from the county courts.
- **Crown Court**—This deals with all serious criminal cases as in England and Wales. Note that terrorist offences are tried in this court without a jury and

they have an automatic right of appeal against both conviction and sentence.

Inferior Courts

- **County courts**—These deal with civil law, including small claims and family cases and are presided over by one of 20 county court judges.
- **District judge (magistrates') courts**—All criminal cases start here and they also deal with a wide range of civil disputes, including Public Health legislation and debt recovery.

SUMMARY

This chapter provides a brief overview of the structure and history of the three current legal systems within the United Kingdom. It defines the categories and sources of law and the jury service. It outlines the judiciary and courts within each legal system, with a summary of the types of case heard in each court and the maximum penalties allowed. It provides simplified flowcharts for the hierarchy of the legal systems in Scotland and in England and Wales, the judiciary in England and Wales and the pathways of criminal procedures and appeals.

USEFUL WEBSITES

English and Welsh Courts: www.judiciary.uk
Scottish Courts: www.scotcourts.gov.uk
Northern Ireland Courts: www.justice-ni.gov.uk

CHAPTER 2

Legal Procedure and Appearing in Court

INTRODUCTION

Any healthcare professional (HCP) with experience in the emergency department is likely to be asked to appear in court at some point in their career. Some HCPs may unfortunately become the subjects of civil litigation for alleged negligence and others may decide to become expert witnesses. There are many good books on the subject for those who decide to become experts (see Further reading) but this chapter aims to make the process less daunting for those for whom appearance in court is a rare event.

THE LEGAL PROFESSION

1. *Legal executives* are lawyers who specialise in a particular area of law. They may have law degrees, but the majority learn their trade through work experience and may gain further qualifications through the Chartered Institute of Legal Executives (CILEx).
2. *Solicitors* qualify through either the Solicitors Qualifying Examination (SQE) or the Legal Practice Course (LPC) route and both also require a 2-year period of 'recognised training'. Most solicitors work in private practice and deal with different aspects of the law such as conveyancing, family law, divorce, wills, estates and business law. Their role in criminal law is to protect and advance the legal rights of the accused. They advise their client and may represent him in lower courts. Solicitors can also take a test to act as an advocate in higher courts.
3. *Barristers* are self-employed and can only be engaged by solicitors, not the public. After gaining the LLB

or the CPE, trainee barristers must take the Bar Vocational Course for a year and then spend a year as a pupil of a senior barrister. Barristers give advice on points of law and procedures and represent their client in court. They are also known as Counsel and wear wigs and gowns.
4. *Judges and Sheriffs*—see Chapter 1.
5. *Coroners and Procurator Fiscals*—see Chapter 11.

PROCEEDINGS AT AN INQUEST OR FATAL ACCIDENT INQUIRY

See Chapter 11.

CIVIL LITIGATION

Civil cases are heard in the county and High Courts in Northern Ireland, and England and Wales and in the Sheriff Courts and the Court of Session in Scotland (see Chapter 1) but the majority settle before going to court. Personal injury cases valued at more than £50,000 can start in the High Courts but most begin in the county or Sheriff Courts, as there is no limit to the damages that they can award. Civil cases are usually heard before a single judge but there is a right of trial before jury in cases alleging slander, libel, malicious prosecution or false imprisonment. Civil litigation is often protracted and expensive but must follow the *Civil Procedure Rules* (CPR) and is now more streamlined following the introduction of the *Legal Aid Sentencing and Punishment of Offenders Act 2013*.

Actions usually begin with the injured party (claimant) consulting a solicitor, who collects information and advises his client if he believes that there is a case to answer. This may include a preliminary report by an expert. The claimant should also consider if the defendant has sufficient assets to fund any likely damages and if it may result in adverse publicity. The solicitor then sends a Letter of Claim, warning the defendant of litigation if settlement is not reached. The defendant is served with a claim form with particulars of the claim and if he fails to respond within 14 days (28 days if they send an acknowledgement), the claimant may be entitled to a judgement by default. If the defendant does respond, then both parties must provide to each other all the key documents relating to the case (disclosure). This is the preaction stage and must be completed under the CPR prior to commencement of proceedings to determine if any early resolution is possible or to ensure a fair trial. The following may then occur:

1. The claimant discontinues his action.
2. The parties reach agreement (settle) before going to court. This may involve arbitration or alternative dispute resolution (ADR) (see later).
3. The court decides there is no defence and a summary judgement is made for the claimant.
4. The defendant obtains a dismissal on the grounds that the claim is weak.
5. The case goes to trial. The burden of proof is on the claimant (see later) and the standard is lower than that of criminal cases in that it is the *balance of probabilities*, i.e. which account is most likely to be the true version of events. The claimant must show:
   a. that the defendant was responsible for his loss or damage (liability)
   b. if liability is established, the amount of damages that are due to compensate him for his loss (quantum) or that other measures, e.g. an injunction, is necessary. Quantum is set either by a standard book or by the jury in jury trials, often following advice from an expert witness.
6. Both parties can appeal the judgement.

Arbitration

This is an adjudication process that operates outside the court, where a third party reviews the case and makes a decision that is binding on both parties. In the county court, it is imposed automatically on defended cases where the claim is less than £1000. It is less formal than court proceedings, although witnesses may be called to give evidence, and it offers a quicker solution, but legal aid is not available. If the claim is for more than £1000, the parties can still opt for arbitration and may choose their own arbitrator.

Alternative Dispute Resolution (ADR)

This is another alternative to civil litigation, where a third party acts as a mediator but his decision is not binding and the disputing parties must negotiate their own settlement. If they cannot reach an agreement, then they may go on to arbitration. This process is useful if the parties wish to retain a working relationship and the court will expect the use of ADR to have been explored, with some limited exceptions, prior to proceedings being commenced.

CRIMINAL PROCEEDINGS

The system used for criminal proceedings in the United Kingdom is adversarial and the burden of proof is on the prosecution, i.e. they must prove that the defendant is guilty by calling evidence to support their case. The defence then tests the evidence and attempts to prove that it is not reliable and does not prove guilt to the required standard. If the defendant mounts a defence, e.g. provocation or self-defence, then the prosecution must also disprove that. The standard of proof is *beyond reasonable doubt*, i.e. the magistrates or the jury must be convinced that the defendant is guilty. Rarely, the evidential burden can shift to the defence if a specific defence is raised, e.g. a plea of insanity or diminished responsibility, but in such cases, the standard is lowered to that of civil proceedings, i.e. the *balance of probabilities*.

The Prosecutor

In England and Wales, the Crown Prosecution Service (CPS) conducts the majority of criminal cases and all police-initiated prosecutions. The CPS was created in 1986 by the *Prosecution of Offences Act 1985* and is headed by the Director of Public Prosecutions (DPP). The CPS engages barristers to conduct the prosecution in the higher courts, but CPS solicitors may act as advocates in the lower courts. The Scottish equivalent is the Crown Office (see Chapter 1) and in the High Court, the Lord Advocate or one of his Deputes conducts the prosecution. In the Sheriff and District Courts, this is done by the local Procurator Fiscal or one of his Deputes. In England and Wales, cases are brought as *R* (Regina) *v N* (name of defendant) and in Scotland, they are *HMA* (Her Majesty's Advocate) *v N*. Other public prosecuting authorities include the Customs and Excise, the Serious Fraud Office and the Inland Revenue. Individuals may also bring private prosecutions, but this is very rare.

The Defendant

The defendant may also be called the accused and if he pleads guilty, then no evidence is called and there is no trial before sentencing. The judge may decide to hear from the prosecution and defence to decide sentencing; this is known as a 'Newton hearing'. If the defendant admits his guilt to his legal representative but then pleads not guilty, he is entitled to a trial to test the evidence to prove his guilt, but he cannot mount a defence.

Children under 10 years (child) cannot be prosecuted as they are presumed incapable of committing criminal acts. They can at age 10 to 14 (young offender) but the prosecution must prove that they committed the offence and that they were aware that what they were doing was wrong. Cases involving young offenders under 18 years in England and Wales must be heard in the Youth or Crown Court but there are no special courts for young offenders in Scotland.

Arrest and Prosecution

Under the *Police and Criminal Evidence Act (PACE) 1984*, a police officer may arrest anyone that he 'on reasonable grounds, suspects is about to, or is in the act of or has committed an arrestable offence'. The person must be told that he is under arrest and given the reasons for it. He must also be reminded of his right to remain silent. However, as the court may now draw an adverse inference from this silence, he must also be cautioned that it may harm his defence if he does not mention when questioned something that he may later rely on in court. The person is then taken to the police station to be charged if there is sufficient evidence, or detained for the purposes of gathering such evidence, including interview on tape. The way the detainee is treated while in the station is strictly regulated under *PACE 1984*. The detainee has certain rights and entitlements, including the right to free independent legal advice, to read the Codes of Practice and to have someone informed of his arrest. The detainee is then:

1. released with no further action (NFA) or a formal warning.
2. charged and released with a caution from the inspector.
3. charged and released with requirement to pay a Fixed Penalty Notice (FPN).
4. released on (un)conditional bail pending further investigation. Following the provisions of the *Policing and Crime Act 2017*, the maximum length of time that can be spent of bail is now 28 days.
5. charged and released on bail as above with a date to appear in court.
6. released under investigation (RUI)—this is similar to bail but has no time limits or conditions.
7. detained for further questioning—for 24 hours initially but this can be extended to 36 hours by a police superintendent or above. An application can also be made to the magistrates' court to allow detention up to 96 hours in total. Suspects arrested under the *Terrorism Act* can be detained under certain conditions for up to 14 days without charge.
8. charged and detained to appear before the magistrates' court if there are reasons that he should not be given bail, e.g. breach of previous bail conditions or no fixed address.

The action taken depends on several factors, including the nature and seriousness of the offence, the circumstances and the degree of intent. The investigating officer prepares the case notes and sends them to the CPS or the Fiscal, who decide whether to prosecute. For serious cases in Scotland, the decision rests with the Crown Counsel and it is based on a report from the Fiscal. In these cases, he must make his own investigations, interview witnesses and gather evidence.

The decision in all cases depends on the following:

1. *Evidential test*—There must be sufficient evidence to provide a 'realistic prospect of conviction'. If not, the CPS or the Fiscal can direct the police to carry out further enquiries or discontinue the case.
2. *Public interest test*—It must be in the public interest and that of the victim to proceed with the case, e.g. use of a weapon or assault on a public servant (e.g. an HCP or police officer).

The defence solicitor can also make representations against prosecution.

The CPS, Crown Office or Fiscal can discontinue a case at any point in the proceedings but if they decide to proceed, details of the charges and the evidence upon which they are based are given to the accused. The Scottish equivalent is a *complaint,* which is served by the Fiscal. The offence with which the accused is charged is important, as it must reflect his conduct and obtain a conviction with adequate sentencing powers. The solicitor then prepares the defence, including interviewing witnesses and instructing experts to counteract those for the prosecution. The nature of the defence and any alibi evidence must be disclosed to the court. There are very strict rules regarding disclosure and these are contained in the *Criminal Procedure and Investigations Act 1996* and *Criminal Procedure (Scotland) Act 1995* (see Chapter 6). In Scotland, more serious cases are set out in a *petition* to the Sheriff, who grants a warrant for the detention of the accused.

In cases where it is not deemed necessary to arrest the offender, e.g. following an investigation by the Inland Revenue, he will be issued with a summons. This advises him that he is believed to have committed an offence and gives him a date to appear in court.

Mode of Trial

This depends on the category of the offence. In England and Wales, there are three categories:

1. *Summary*—These may only be heard in the magistrates' court, e.g. common assault, minor driving infractions.
2. *Indictable*—These can only be tried before the Crown Court, e.g. rape, murder, but they first appear

in the magistrates' court for a committal hearing. This allows the magistrates to decide if there is sufficient reliable evidence to allow the jury to convict, i.e. to act as a filter.

3. *Either way*—These can heard in the Crown Court or the magistrates' court and the decision is made at a mode of trial hearing, where the magistrates hear representations from both the prosecution and the defence. Defendants can request a Crown Court hearing, but not magistrates'. If the decision is made for a Crown Court hearing, the case goes before a committal hearing as for (2).

Note that the magistrates' court also decides if the accused should:

- be released on bail or remanded in custody to await trial
- receive legal aid—this is based on both a means test and whether it is in the public interest for him to receive it.

In Scotland, the categories are the following:

1. *Summary*—These are dealt with by the Fiscal and are heard before the Sheriff Court.

2. *Solemn*—These are more serious cases and are heard initially in the Sheriff Court for a judicial examination, where the accused can answer the allegations and the prosecution can cross-examine him. The accused must then either be released on bail or remanded to custody (if accused of treason, murder or if the Crown objects to bail). If he is held in custody, the prosecution must serve him with an indictment, outlining the allegations, list of witnesses and evidence within 80 days or he must be released. Trials of less serious cases are also heard in the Sheriff Court before a jury, but the Sheriff can refer the case to the High Court for sentencing. Very serious cases, e.g. rape or murder, are heard before the High Court.

Seating arrangements

- The judge/sheriff/magistrate/Justice of the Peace sits at the head of the courtroom on a raised platform, commonly known as the Bench.
- The Clerk of Court sits in front of the Bench and is often accompanied by the stenographer.
- Counsels for the prosecution and defence sit facing the Bench, with their instructing solicitors or representative from the CPS sitting behind them. Defence counsel usually sits at the side closest to the jury, but this varies.
- The jury sits to the side of the Bench, usually on the right.

- The defendant sits facing the Bench, behind the prosecutor in an area commonly known as the Dock.
- Witnesses stand on a raised platform known as the witness box or wait outside until the Usher calls them. In Scotland, the equivalent to the Usher is the Court Officer or Macer (High Court).
- Members of the public sit in the public gallery, which is usually at the rear of the court.

Order of proceedings

In the magistrates' court, the case is tried before a 'bench' of three lay justices or one district judge. They are responsible for reaching the verdict and sentencing where necessary. In a Crown Court, the trial takes place before a judge and jury. The jury decides the verdict, but the judge has responsibility for the sentencing. The judge may only question the witness to clarify a point and may not cross-examine. In Scotland, cases are heard in the High Court by a judge and jury as for the Crown Court. In the Sheriff Court, there is one Sheriff (with a jury in more serious cases) and in the District Court, there is usually one Justice of the Peace but there may be more. The prosecutor in England and Wales is the counsel for the CPS for all courts. In Scotland, High Court cases are prosecuted by an Advocate Depute and Sheriff Court cases by the Procurator Fiscal. The order is the same in the civil courts, but the counsel for the claimant replaces the prosecutor.

1. Where present, the jury is sworn in.
2. The charge is read to the defendant and he is asked whether he pleads guilty or not guilty.
3. If the defendant pleads not guilty, the prosecutor makes his opening speech to outline his case (not Scotland).
4. The prosecutor calls and questions the witnesses for the prosecution. This is known as 'examination in chief'.
5. The defence may cross-examine each witness, either to undermine the evidence or to elicit other, more favourable evidence.
6. The prosecutor can then reexamine each witness but for the purposes of clarification only—he may not introduce new topics.
7. The defence may then make a submission of no case to answer—usually on the basis that there is insufficient evidence or that it has been so discredited that a reasonable tribunal would not convict.
8. The prosecutor has a right of reply.
9. If the submission succeeds, the defendant is acquitted.

10. The defence may (but rarely does) make an opening speech.
11. The defence calls and questions the witnesses for the defence.
12. The prosecutor may cross-examine each witness as for (4).
13. The defence may reexamine each witness as for (5).
14. The prosecutor may be allowed to call rebuttal evidence.
15. The prosecutor makes a closing speech (except in the magistrates' court).
16. The defence may make a closing speech if he did not make an opening one.
17. The judge or Sheriff sums up the facts and the law to the jury if present.
18. The jury or magistrates give their verdict. Note:
    - In England and Wales, the jury verdict should be unanimous, although a majority verdict of 10:2 may be accepted if the jury cannot reach agreement after a second period of deliberation. In Scotland, the jury verdict is by a simple majority of at least eight.
    - In England and Wales, the verdict can only be guilty or not guilty. In Scotland, there is a third option of 'not proven', where the accused is acquitted but has not been proved innocent.
19. The judge, sheriff or magistrates decides sentence. This may occur now or at a later date after the judge has received reports. Some offences carry statutory sentences, others depend on the discretion of the judge and may be influenced by factors such as past offences, mitigating circumstances and time already spent in custody.

Evidence
- There must be sufficient evidence to prove the case for the prosecution.
- Evidence can be oral, written or in the form of objects.
- Only 'facts in issue' and evidence relevant to them (circumstantial) are admissible, e.g. for a rape case, the 'facts in issue' are the following:
  1. Sexual intercourse must have occurred (*actus reus* = the act).
  2. The accused must have known or was 'reckless' to the fact that it was without consent (*mens rea* = the intention).
- The circumstantial evidence could include DNA and semen samples.
- Direct evidence is that which requires no mental processing by the judge or jury, e.g. an eye-witness account.

- Circumstantial evidence requires the judge or jury to draw inferences, e.g. motive, opportunity or fingerprints.
- Hearsay evidence is reported speech, e.g. witness statements.

Witnesses
There are three types of witness:
1. *Witness of fact*—He gives factual evidence, i.e. what he heard, saw or read. He is not paid but may claim his travelling expenses.
2. *Professional witness*—He also provides factual evidence but can give some opinions. He usually gives evidence relating to something has seen in the course of his job, e.g. ED doctor. He is paid a fee related to the time that he has been in court and travelling expenses.
3. *Expert witness*—He provides both fact and opinion evidence. His role is to guide the court over matters that are the subject of special expertise.

As an HCP, you can be required to appear as any type of witness, e.g. in a case where the defendant has been alleged to have committed actual bodily harm, you may be a:
1. *Witness of fact*—If you saw the act committed.
2. *Professional witness*—If you treated the victim for his injuries.
3. *Expert witness*—If you are an expert in the causation of different types of injury.

APPEARING IN COURT
Requirement to Attend
Criminal cases
You should receive a letter from the relevant Criminal Justice Unit (CJU) or Fiscal's office, giving you the court and the time and date(s) on which the case is due to be heard. You will be given the name of the defendant but, as it is most likely that you will have seen the victim, you may have to contact the CJU or Fiscal so that you can obtain the relevant notes and read your copy of your statement (see Chapter 4). You will be asked to confirm in writing that you will be available to attend. If you do not reply or refuse to attend without good reason, the prosecution and/or defence can apply to the court for a witness summons or citation (Scotland). This is a written order, which is served on you personally and demands your attendance. If you ignore the order, you risk being arrested and taken to court where you may be fined and/or imprisoned. The CJU or Fiscal's office will usually telephone you the night before the hearing to confirm the time and the court number.

You can ask them if they are prepared to take a contact telephone number and to ring you only if you are actually needed to attend. Cases are often postponed or dismissed at very short notice, or it may be agreed that your statement can be read to the court (this is called 'Section 9'), making your attendance unnecessary. If you do make this request, remember that it is solely for your convenience so you must be easily available and able to get to the court with the minimum of delay.

Civil cases
Your instructing solicitors will usually ask you if you are willing to attend voluntarily. If you refuse or do not reply, they can obtain a witness summons as outlined earlier.

Preparation for Court
- If it is possible, familiarise yourself with the court layout—preferably by visiting it prior to your date of attendance.
- Attend a training course on giving evidence.
- Practice giving evidence in front of colleagues and ask for feedback.
- Decide in advance the strong points in your evidence, i.e. those that the judge, jury or magistrates need to know to make a reasoned decision. These are your strengths and you should return to them as often as possible, even if the question does not really relate to them. This is particularly important if you are an expert witness.
- Dress smartly, conservatively and cover any visible tattoos—remember that the magistrates or jury do not know you and will judge both you and your evidence by your appearance.
- Bring your contemporaneous notes and any relevant X-rays, photographs, etc. with you as:
  a. You can refer to them while giving your evidence although if you do, the opposing party has a right to see them.
  b. If you do not bring them, you can be sent back to retrieve them, which is both humiliating and time-consuming.
- Bring a copy of your statement. You will not be allowed to refer to it in court, but you should read it again before you go in.
- If you are an expert witness, bring a clean copy of your report. You will be allowed to refer to it in court but only if there are no annotations.

Arrival at Court
- Arrive slightly early as counsel may wish to talk to you before you give your evidence.

- Give the Witness Service your name and that of the trial for which you are a witness.
- Ask the CPS or Fiscal's office for a copy of your statement if you do not have one.
- Ask the Usher how you should address the judge or magistrate or use the table shown.
- If you are appearing as a professional witness or a witness to fact, you will not be allowed to enter the courtroom before you give evidence and will be directed to the waiting area. If you are an expert witness, you will usually be allowed to sit in the court in England and Wales but only with the leave of the court in Scotland.

Giving Evidence
See Table 2.1.

Criminal cases
- On entering the witness box, you will be sworn in. You will be asked by the Court Usher (or the Judge in Scotland) if you wish to swear on the bible or other holy book or to give the oath of affirmation.
  Remember that the penalties for perjury (lying while under oath) are severe!
- You must give your evidence orally unless the opposing party agrees that your written statement can be read out, i.e. they do not wish to cross-examine you on what you have written.
- You will then be asked your name, current post, qualifications and relevant experience. It is useful to memorise the first paragraph of your statement (see Chapter 4), as it looks more impressive to provide the information as a whole without being asked for it piecemeal. Remember that you are trying to convince the jury or magistrates that you are a professional person with sufficient qualifications and experience to make your evidence valid, reliable and significant. Do not use abbreviations—give your qualifications their full title, source and the date on which you obtained them, e.g. 'I obtained the FRCS, which is the Fellowship of the Royal College of Surgeons in London in 1993'.
- Speak slowly, clearly and loudly enough for the judge and jury to hear you easily. Use everyday language or the judge or counsel will constantly interrupt your train of thought to ask you to explain what you mean.
- Remember to ask the judge if you can refer to your notes—they almost invariably agree but you must ask.
- Your own counsel will examine you—usually by taking you through your statement or expert report.

TABLE 2.1
Correct Forms of Address

Court	Who Sits?	What Do I Call Them?
ENGLAND AND WALES		
Northern Ireland		
Magistrates' court	Magistrate	'Sir' or 'Madam'
	Justice of Peace	'Sir' or 'Madam'
Crown Court	Circuit judge	'Your Honour'
	Recorder	'Your Honour'
	High Court judge	'Your Lordship/Ladyship' or 'My Lord/Lady'
County court	District judge	'Sir' or 'Madam'
	Circuit judge	'Your Honour'
High Court	High Court judge	'Your Lordship/Ladyship' or 'My Lord/Lady'
Court of Appeal	Lord Chief Justice	'Your Lordship/Ladyship' or 'My Lord/Lady'
Supreme Court	Lords of Appeal	'Your Lordship/Ladyship' or 'My Lord/Lady'
Coroner's Court	Coroner	'Sir' or 'Madam'
SCOTLAND		
District Court	Justice of Peace	'Your Honour'
Sheriff Court	Sheriff	'Your Lordship/Ladyship' or 'My Lord/Lady'
Court of Session	Lords Ordinary	'Your Lordship/Ladyship' or 'My Lord/Lady'
High Court of Justiciary	Lord Commissioners of Judiciary	'Your Lordship/Ladyship' or 'My Lord/Lady'
Fiscal Court	Procurator Fiscal	'Procurator Fiscal' or 'Sir' or 'Madam'

- You will then be cross-examined by the opposing counsel. Remember it is his job to introduce reasonable doubt so he may try to discredit both you and your evidence. It is very difficult not to take this personally, but you should think of it as a compliment that he considers your evidence to be so crucial to the case!
- Do not be concerned if you have to keep repeating your answer—barristers will frequently ask the same question, phrased in different ways in the hope of eliciting new or different information.
- **Never** volunteer information!
- Use the questions to return to the strengths of your evidence.
- You may then be reexamined by your own counsel, but only for the purposes of clarification.
- You must address your answers to the jury or magistrates so stand facing them, turn to face counsel when he asks you a question, then turn back. This technique also makes it more difficult for counsel to interrupt you.
- The judge can only ask you questions to clarify a point and you must answer him directly.

- If counsel asks you a question that you do not understand, is unclear or too convoluted, you can appeal to the judge for clarification. Refer to the barrister as 'counsel'. The judge will then ask him to either rephrase the question or withdraw it unless he feels that it was a fair question, in which case he will direct you to answer it.
- Never speak directly to the barrister or argue with him—you will lose!
- Remember that as a witness of fact, you cannot give opinions.
- As a professional witness, you may be asked for your opinion but take care not to stray out of your field of expertise—it is far better to admit that you do not know something than made to appear to be a liar or ignorant.
- If you are an expert witness, then you have been called specifically to give evidence of both fact and opinion:
  a. Your factual evidence has two parts and you must clearly identify the source:
     i. Your own observations, e.g. if you have been asked to examine the victim of an assault.

   ii. The facts that you have been told in order to prepare your report, e.g. a copy of the original ED notes.
b. Your opinion evidence involves the conclusions that you have reached using your specialist expertise and experience after considering the facts.
c. Remember that your report is privileged, i.e. accessible only by the instructing solicitor and his client and if the solicitor feels that it might be prejudicial to his client's case, he can conceal it. However, if the solicitor does decide to use it at trial, then it must be revealed to the other side at disclosure and the privilege is lost. Note that privilege applies **only** to reports prepared for litigation purposes.
d. The opposing party will have had access to your report early in the case so be prepared for some rigorous cross-examination.
- Remember that Part 35 of the *Civil Procedure Rules 1998* states that your role as an expert witness is to help the court and this overrides any obligation to the party paying you.

Civil cases
- The process is essentially the same.
- The claimant's case is heard first.
- If the defendant is insured, his insurance company will usually run his case. For an HCP, it will be run by either the Trust solicitors or his defence society. For a hospital or Trust, it will be run by the Trust solicitors (see Chapter 9).
- If you are an expert witness, you will probably be asked for your opinion on both liability and quantum to assist the judge in his final decision.

After Giving Evidence
- Stay in the witness box until you are given leave by the judge.

- Check that you are released from court. You may be asked to remain in court to hear subsequent evidence, advise counsel on opposing medical opinion or be recalled to give further evidence.
- If you have appeared as a professional witness, make sure that you have been given a claim form, as you are entitled to a fee and your travelling expenses, whether you have given evidence or not.
- If you are an expert witness, you should negotiate your fee with the solicitor before accepting his instructions and have it confirmed in writing. If the case is legally aided, then you must complete a claim form from the Crown Court office.

SUMMARY
This chapter allows the reader to understand the structure of the legal profession. It also explains how civil and criminal cases arise and how they proceed both before and during court proceedings. It provides a clear picture of what to expect, the legal obligations and how to behave if the reader is called as a witness in court, from the initial request to giving evidence.

FURTHER READING
Bond, C., Solon, M., Harper, P., Davies, G. *The expert witness: a practical guide*. Crayford: Shaw and Sons Ltd; 2007.

USEFUL WEBSITES
English and Welsh Courts: www.gov.uk/government/organisations/hm-court-service
Scottish Courts: www.scotcourts.gov.uk
Northern Ireland Courts: www.justice-ni.gov.uk
GMC Guidance: www.gmc-uk.org/ethical-guidance/ethical-guidance-for-doctors/acting as a witness

CHAPTER 3

Preparing a Police Statement

BOX 3.1
Statements

- Accurate
- Legible
- Complete
- Impartial
- Understandable
- Based on fact, not opinion

THE PURPOSE OF A STATEMENT

In the majority of cases where you have been asked to provide a statement, you will have seen the alleged victim of an assault. There is no legal obligation to complete a statement, but there is an ethical and, for some healthcare professionals (HCPs), e.g. Forensic Medical Examiners (FMEs) or Custody Nurse Practitioners (CNPs), a contractual obligation to do so. In criminal cases, statements are made under Section 9 of the *Criminal Justice Act 1967*, the *Criminal Procedure Rules*, Section 102 of the *Magistrates Courts Act 1980* and rule 90 of the *Magistrates Courts Rules 1981*. Statements made in Scotland and Northern Ireland can be read in the same way as those taken in England and Wales, provided all the provisions of Section 9 of the *Criminal Justice Act 1967* have been complied with, but not statements from outside the United Kingdom. Your statement will be required to:

- inform the investigating officer of your findings and any treatment given
- form the basis of your factual evidence as a professional witness
- be used by the prosecuting counsel as a guide for his examination-in-chief
- be used by the defence counsel as a guide for his cross-examination
- confirm the chain of evidence in relation to forensic samples and examples (see Chapter 4).

It is very important that all statements are completed at the same time that they are requested, as the case may be unnecessarily delayed if not.

WRITING A STATEMENT
General Principles

The same rules should apply to a statement as writing clinical notes. A statement should be everything listed in Box 3.1:

BOX 3.2
Essential Paragraph

'This statement, consisting of x pages, each signed by me, is true to the best of my knowledge and belief, and I make it knowing that, if it is tendered in evidence, I shall be liable to prosecution if I have wilfully stated in it anything which I know to be false or do not believe to be true'.

For obvious reasons, a typewritten statement is vastly superior but if it must be written by hand, it is essential that it is legible. Any errors should be corrected manually by a single line drawn through in ink and initialled. NEVER use correction fluid as this may lead to allegations that the statement has been altered to the detriment of either the accused or the victim!

The police supply form MG11 for statements in England and Wales or 38/36 in Northern Ireland, but it is not mandatory nor is it necessary to have your signature witnessed. If you have a computer, you may find it useful to design your own template, but it must contain the paragraph shown in Box 3.2.

Writing a Statement on Behalf of Someone Else

If the investigating officer is unable to contact the HCP who saw the victim of an alleged assault, he may ask you to write a statement based on the notes made at the time. This is obviously not an ideal situation and many HCPs do not feel able to provide such a statement. However, this may mean that the police cannot pursue the case, as they do not have written evidence of any injuries and this would be unfair to the alleged victim. There should be no adverse sequelae to making

---

BOX 3.3
Necessary Paragraph

'The medical notes were created or received by (name of examining doctor) in the course of his medical profession and the information contained in the notes was supplied by (name of examining doctor) who had or reasonably supposed to have had personal knowledge of the matters dealt with therein.

Dr (name) is unable to make a statement as ....'

---

a statement based on the notes of another HCP as long as it is made clear that you never saw the patient yourself and that the quality and extent of the statement is entirely dependent on that of the original notes. It is actually documentary hearsay and can only be made admissible as evidence under the *Criminal Justice Act 2003* by the inclusion of the shown in Box 3.3.

CONTENT

Your statement should contain the following:

Your Employment and Qualifications

Always start a statement with a paragraph about you: your name, grade or post, place of employment, your qualifications and from where they were obtained. If you do have any specialist knowledge relevant to the case, this should also be noted. This paragraph gives your statement credibility and makes it less likely that you will be asked to appear in court.

The Patient's Name and Age

Always state the name and age of your patient so there is no possibility of mistaken identity. Never include either your own or the patients' address! The opposing side may see your statement.

Day, Date, Time and Place of Your Examination

Be specific about writing the day, date, time and place of your examination so there can be no confusion. Use the 24-hour clock at all times and state the name and role of anyone else present, e.g. a chaperone or relative.

Consent

You should state that you obtained *informed voluntary* consent from the patient for both the examination and preparation of the statement (see Chapter 5). **Never** write a statement unless you have seen written confirmation that the patient agrees to disclosure of the clinical notes. This should be attached to the request for the statement. Consent for examination is less important as consent can be implied from the fact that the patient came to see you for treatment (see Chapter 5).

The Reason for the Examination

Give the reason why you examined this patient. It is particularly important to note whether this was solely for treatment of injuries sustained or whether there was a forensic element to the examination. Some patients will present to you purely for documentation of their injuries and may have only come because they have been advised to do so by the police.

Any Reported History

Although this is hearsay evidence (see Chapter 2), it is often useful with regard to explaining the reason for the examination and your findings. Every assault is alleged until proved otherwise, but a statement such *as* 'Mr X told me that he had been hit with a hammer but only on the head' incriminates no one while explaining why you only examined his head.

Full Details of Your Findings

Write everything in your statement that you wrote in your notes but use lay terms wherever possible. Remember that it is unlikely that either the investigating officer or the judge will be medically qualified and you do not want to put yourself in the position of being called to court merely to explain what you meant by an obscure medical term. Negative findings are often as important as the positive in statements, as they may refute a false allegation. Remember to measure wounds and give those measurements (see Description of injuries). Unless you are an expert, you are not allowed to express an opinion in court regarding causality so do not give one in your statement. If you offer an opinion, you risk being discredited in court when opposing counsel asks you about your previous experience, qualifications and the background upon which you based your inference. The investigating officer may ask you what you think but you are legally not obliged to answer nor should you. Never give an opinion as to the possible cause of the injury or the likely weapon even if requested to do so.

Forensic Samples

List any forensic samples as shown in Chapter 4.

Any Treatment Given

Investigating officers are often very interested in the type of treatment that a victim required, as it can give them some indication of the severity of the injuries sustained. To a lay person, a patient who required admission would appear to be more severely injured than one who could be discharged with analgesics and this can impress a judge or jury more than lengthy descriptions of the actual injuries. The type of injury will also influence the charge and can change 'actual bodily harm' to 'grievous bodily harm' (see Chapter 14). This has far-reaching consequences for the final sentence handed down.

Sign the Statement

This is possibly the most important part of writing a statement, as an unsigned statement is inadmissible in court. Note that this first page must be signed twice and each subsequent page must also be signed. The signature does not need to be witnessed.

Complete the Reverse of the Statement Form

The reverse of form MG11 asks for contact details and dates to be avoided. Never give your home address or telephone number, but it is helpful to give the hospital or practice address and telephone number. It is also useful to give any dates when you know you will not be available, e.g. holidays, although you will be asked to provide these details again if the case goes to court. Note that this side is not included when the statement is copied for the defence lawyers.

Take a Copy

Make sure that you retain a copy of the statement for your own records. Cases may come to court months or even years later and although the police should provide you with a copy, it is useful to keep your own. It should be kept in a secure place and if it is a computerised record, it should be kept at your place of employment, as it is then subject to GDPR (see Chapter 6).

Complete the Fee Note

Complete the fee note and take a copy, as it is your only record of when you completed the statement and to whom it was sent. There is a statutory fee for each statement provided, but there are often delays in payment and you may need to pursue the police station involved. Remember that you will be expected to pay tax on all fees received so be sure to keep accurate records.

DESCRIPTION OF INJURIES

When recording injuries in your clinical notes, it is beneficial to draw a diagram in order to precisely record the site of the injury. This is particularly important

---

> **BOX 3.4**
> **Recording Injuries**
>
> 1. Group descriptions according to anatomical site and note the number at each site
> 2. Describe the position of wounds in relation to fixed anatomical points
> 3. Describe the colour and shape of all injuries
> 4. Accurately measure all injuries
> 5. Use the correct descriptive term for each injury

when there are multiple injuries, but if you refer to any diagrams in your statement, they have to be produced as exhibits using your initials followed by consecutive numbers, e.g. 'VGM/1'. You might prefer to describe the injuries in text form and this will be made easier and more accurate by applying the rules shown in Box 3.4 when writing both your notes and statements.

Group Descriptions According to Anatomical Site

Ideally, injuries should be documented in a sequential order, starting at the head and working distally to the feet. Injuries should be grouped, e.g. all injuries to the right arm should be described together even if they are different types of injury. Record the number of injuries so there is no confusion and no injuries are missed.

Describe the Position of Wounds in Relation to Fixed Anatomical Points

The position of a wound should be related to a fixed anatomical point such as the elbow, knee or umbilicus. This allows the wound to be more accurately documented—e.g. 'an incised wound on the forearm 10 cm from the elbow on the palmar surface'. Be particularly stringent while looking for defence wounds. These include cuts on the hands, especially between the fingers and over the palms, and an isolated transverse fracture of the ulna.

Accurately Measure All Injuries

All injuries should be accurately measured using a ruler or measuring tape. Metric units are the system of choice, but imperial can be used. It is more important that the system used is consistent throughout the documentation.

Describe the Colour and Shape of All Injuries

Never try to age bruises. There have been many publications on the subject, but visual ageing of bruising remains an inexact science. The most that can be said is that a bruise with any degree of yellowing is almost certainly at least 18 hours old.[1] It is essential to record any active bleeding and whether there are any signs of healing. A moist wound is likely to have occurred some time in the preceding 24 hours whereas a scabbed wound is probably older. Shape is best described as simply as possible, e.g. *crescentic, V-shaped or irregular*.

Use the Correct Descriptive Term for Each Injury

The following are all terms that have both legal and forensic significance. If you are forced to use a specialised medical term, you must try to explain what it means but it is better to use lay terms wherever possible for the reasons given earlier (Table 3.1).

Erythema or redness

Erythema is caused by pressure and can be patterned, reflecting the overlying clothing. It disappears after about 24 hours and may warrant a photograph, especially if it outlines an apparent injury such as the imprint of a hand.

Petechiae

Petechiae are caused by arteriolar rupture and are pinpoint haemorrhages <2 mm in diameter. They are associated with congestion and asphyxia so are commonly found in the head and neck of victims who have suffered a strangulation attempt. Petechiae are most easily seen in the mouth and the eyes where they may be associated with retinal and subconjunctival haemorrhages. They may also be caused by suction and the characteristic 'love-bite' is actually a collection of petechiae.

Abrasion or graze or scratch

Although clinically only a minor wound, abrasions can have enormous forensic significance, particularly where the victim is dead. Abrasions are superficial skin injuries that do not penetrate the full thickness of the epidermis, although they may bleed due to corrugations of the dermal papillae. They are caused

TABLE 3.1
Terms of Legal and Forensic Significance

Medical Term	Lay Term
Erythema	Redness
Petechiae	
Abrasion	Graze or scratch
Contusion	Bruise
Haematoma	
Laceration	Burst wound
Incised wound	Stab or puncture
Slash or cut	Slash or cut
Periorbital haematoma	Black eye
Bite	Bite

by a tangential dragging or frictional force so the end opposite to the point of impact shows heaped-up epidermis. This means that the direction of force can be deduced, e.g. for victims of hit-and-run accidents (Fig. 3.1).

Contusion or bruise

Bruises are subcutaneous haemorrhages and they are caused by a blunt force. Like erythema, they can be patterned and may reproduce the weapon responsible, e.g. the sole of a shoe. However, the bleeding may track under the skin, leading to confluence and loss of the pattern. It is important to note that the size of the bruise does not necessarily reflect the degree of force applied nor the size of the object used to inflict it. Bruises tend to be larger where the skin is lax or if there is underlying bone and there may be no bruising at all in areas where the skin is thick or closely applied to the underlying tissues such as the palm or the soles of the feet. This is the principle behind a form of torture used in Turkey called 'Falaka' where the soles of the feet are beaten with sticks. It is excruciatingly painful yet leaves barely a mark. The amount of bruising is also affected by other factors such as age, sex, concurrent illnesses and bleeding diatheses. Patterns of bruising

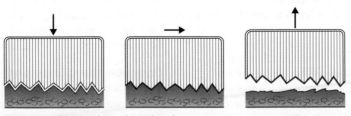

FIG. 3.1 Mechanism of an abrasion.

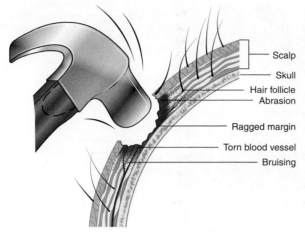

FIG. 3.2 Mechanism of a laceration.

Scalp
Skull
Hair follicle
Abrasion
Ragged margin
Torn blood vessel
Bruising

TABLE 3.2 Differences Between a Laceration and an Incised Wound		
	Laceration	**Incised Wound**
Cause	Blunt force	Sharp object
Edges	Ragged and irregular	Clean and straight
Bruising?	Yes	No
Abrasions?	Yes	No
Depth	Variable	Usually uniform
Tissue bridges?	Yes	No
Position	Usually bony prominences	Anywhere
Foreign bodies?	Frequent— often dirty	Usually clean unless caused by glass

are often more significant, e.g. fingertip bruises. These are circular or oval bruises 1 to 2 cm in diameter and they are classically found over the limbs or neck where they denote that a gripping force has been applied (see Chapter 14). It is important to distinguish bruising from other innocent causes of skin discoloration such as blue naevi, Campbell de Morgan spots and cyanosis.

Haematoma

This term is often thought to be synonymous with 'bruise', but they are not the same. A haematoma is a palpable collection of blood, usually in muscle, that may require surgical drainage.

Laceration or burst wound

This is probably the most erroneously used medical term of all. A laceration is a full-thickness tear in the skin caused by a perpendicular *blunt* force—it is *not* the same as a cut or incised wound as shown in Table 3.2.

Lacerations are most commonly found over bony prominences such as the scalp, eyebrow or elbows and they are gaping, irregular wounds, often with associated bruising or grazing. They can be linear and may only be differentiated from an incised wound by the edges. Lacerations are often dirty wounds, but their most striking feature is the presence of tissue bridges. These occur because lacerations vary in depth, so some elements of the subcutaneous tissue are left intact whereas others are not. The shape of a laceration may indicate the agent responsible, e.g. hammers cause crescentic wounds. They are rarely self-inflicted, as they are so painful (Fig. 3.2).

Incised wound

Incised wounds can be subdivided into stab or puncture wounds and cuts or slash wounds. A stab wound is deeper than it is long whereas a slash wound is longer than it is deep. Incised wounds are usually clean, linear and of uniform depth. They are caused by sharp objects and the shape of a stab wound can sometimes give an indication of the type of object used to inflict it, although the appearance also depends on other features such as the direction of skin tension. Slash wounds rarely reproduce the dimensions of the weapon well. Annotation of the site of an incised wound is vital as, unlike lacerations, incised wounds can be self-inflicted to support a false allegation. Multiple, superficial slash wounds in easily accessible areas on the opposite side to the dominant hand are especially suspicious, particularly in the presence of old similar scars and a psychiatric history (Fig. 3.3).

Bite

Bites vary from being classic crescentic wounds with either a central pallor or petechiae (indicating sucking) and tooth marks to unremarkable bruises. It is very important to note the position, shape and size as these points can distinguish a human bite from animal and adult from child in abuse cases.

Firearm injuries

Firearm injuries can be subdivided by either the type of missile or the type of weapon:
- **Missile:** There are two types—high (faster than the speed of sound) and low velocity (slower).

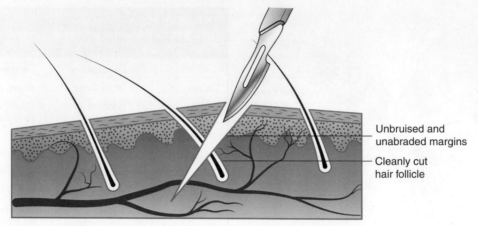

Unbruised and unabraded margins

Cleanly cut hair follicle

FIG. 3.3   Mechanism of an incised wound.

1. *High-velocity missiles*, e.g. from a rifle, cause a permanent cavity but the high-energy transfer also causes surrounding cavitation with ischaemia and visceral rupture. All missile wounds are contaminated but high-energy transfer wounds require more aggressive debridement and they are particularly susceptible to anaerobic infection.
2. *Low-velocity missiles*, e.g. from a handgun, also cause a permanent cavity through crushing and laceration but the damage is limited to the wound track. Such injuries are only fatal if a vital organ is damaged.
- **Weapon**: There are also essentially two types: smooth bore and rifled.
  1. *Smooth-bore weapons* include shotguns and they fire small pellets that emerge as a solid mass then disperse. The resultant wound depends on the distance of the body from the muzzle of the gun. Contact wounds are usually circular with surrounding bruising, laceration and blackening from smoke. As the distance increases, the central wound size becomes smaller with surrounding satellite puncture wounds. Exit wounds are rare.
  2. *Rifled weapons* include revolvers, rifles and pistols. They have parallel spiral ridges inside the barrel that cause the bullet to spin, giving it a straight flight path and characteristic scratches that are unique to each gun. The entry wounds are usually neat round holes, unless the bullet strikes at an angle, with a surrounding abrasion. Contact wounds may also show charring. Exit wounds are usually much larger, with everted, lacerated margins. Note that the calibre of the bullet cannot be judged by the size of the wound.

SUMMARY

This chapter makes the reader aware of the obligations that follow a request to provide a statement to the police and how to accurately prepare and submit such a statement, also called the MG11. It identifies a method for precisely recording injuries and explains how to differentiate between the different types of injury. It also provides a description of the appearance and likely causality of all of the injuries most commonly encountered in healthcare practice.

CASE SCENARIOS

1. During your shift in the emergency department, you were asked to see a 20-year-old woman with injuries to her left forearm. She is distressed and accompanied by a police officer. She says that her partner tried to hit her with a hammer and her arm was injured as she tried to fend him off. Her partner is now under arrest.

   On examination, you find multiple parallel superficial slash wounds with no bruising or swelling and there is no bony tenderness. Is her story consistent with the injuries and what other factors in the history and examination are important?
2. You tell the patient that you cannot find any injuries consistent with hammer blows and she changes her story to one that he tried to stab her with a knife. Is this more likely?
3. You receive a request for a statement by the police, but what can you be sure of before completing and returning it?
4. You receive a letter from the Crown Prosecution Service requesting your attendance at court. Do

you have to go and can you be represented by your medical indemnity provider?

5. While you are being questioned as a professional witness at court, counsel asks you for your 'expert opinion' as to what caused the injury—what should you say?

See 'Answers to case scenarios'.

NOTE

1. Langlois NEI, Gresham GA. The ageing of bruises: a review & study of the colour changes with time. *Forensic Sci Int*. 1991;50:227–238.

FURTHER READING

Payne-James J, Jones RM. *Simpson's forensic medicine*. 14th edn. Boca Raton: CRC Press; 2019.

McLay WDS. *Clinical forensic medicine*. 3rd edn. Cambridge: Cambridge University Press; 2009.

USEFUL WEBSITES

Faculty of Forensic and Legal Medicine: www.fflm.ac.uk
Crown Prosecution Service: www.cps.gov.uk

Forensic Samples

INTRODUCTION

Forensic samples can prove vital to the final outcome of a case but the quality of the evidence that they provide depends on both their collection and analysis. Anything below the highest standard can lead to miscarriages of justice, such as the case of the Birmingham Six[1] where the convictions were based on prosecution evidence that traces of nitroglycerine had been found on the accused. The tests were done using the now-defunct Griess test and the possibility of innocent contamination was not considered. The Birmingham Six were jailed in 1975 and their convictions were not quashed until 1991 so they suffered 16 years of wrongful imprisonment.

This chapter will focus on the collection of forensic samples, as this is the area that can involve the healthcare professional (HCP). Under the current provisions of the *Police and Criminal Evidence Act (PACE) 1984*, the *Prisoners and Criminal Proceedings (Scotland) Act 1993* and the *Road Traffic Act 1988*, intimate samples can only be taken by 'a registered medical practitioner' or 'a registered HCP'. Intimate samples are the following:

- blood, semen or any other tissue fluid
- pubic hair
- swabs from the genital area or all orifices other than the mouth
- dental impressions (can only be taken by registered forensic dentists).

USES OF SAMPLES
DNA Profiling

DNA profiling was introduced in 1986 using the multilocus probe (MLP) technique, which was a significant advance on the conventional blood grouping techniques. MLP was highly discriminating but poorly sensitive, requiring relatively large amounts of chromosomal DNA and it was replaced by the single locus probe (SLP) method, which was more sensitive and could be used on smaller amounts of material. However, SLP was less discriminating and it was often necessary to combine the results of several independent SLPs. In 1994 the Forensic Science Service (FSS) launched a new method of DNA profiling based on the polymerase chain reaction (PCR) technique, whereby a targeted area of DNA can be induced to clone itself by controlled cycles of heating and cooling. This method of DNA profiling analyses areas of DNA called short tandem repeats (STRs). The level of discrimination has now risen to the chance of a random match being less than one in several million and STR results can be obtained from minute amounts of chromosomal DNA, e.g. saliva on envelope seals.

In 1995 the national DNA database was established and changes to *PACE 1984* meant that buccal swabs could be taken by police officers without consent from any detainee charged with a recordable offence. In 2020 the database had 6.6 million profiles, which allowing for duplicates, equates to 5.6 million individuals and it is now run by the Home Office. The UK police services own the profile records on the database and are notified of any matches, but they do not have access to it. All samples that are suitable for DNA profiling from both suspects and crime scenes are submitted for analysis and inclusion in the database. Suspect DNA is cross-referenced against all known crime scenes and vice versa in a continuous process. This not only links suspects to different crimes but may also reveal serial cases, as it can link crimes committed by the same person, even if that person is not yet on the database. A more recent innovation is that of familial searches, where the suspect's DNA profile is matched to one or more relatives on the database but concerns have been raised over confidentiality, as it could lead to the police identifying disputes over paternity.

Initially, the database only held DNA from people who had been convicted of a crime, but the *Criminal Justice and Police Act 2001* allowed DNA to be retained from those who had been charged but not yet convicted and in 2004, the *Criminal Justice Act 2003* extended this further to allow DNA to be taken and stored from anyone who had been arrested for a 'recordable offence'. These profiles were initially retained indefinitely, even if the person was then either not charged or later acquitted but in 2012, the *Protection of Freedoms Act 2012* allowed such people to apply to have their profiles deleted. The DNA Database for Scotland is housed at the Police Forensic Science Laboratory in Dundee and shares its data with the National Database.

DNA profiling has also been used in paternity suits, issues of probate, cases of alleged incest and in the identification of human remains. Analysis of mitochondrial DNA has extended DNA profiling to an even wider range of material, including hair shafts.

Biochemical Analysis

- Hair and other objects, e.g. fibres retrieved from the victim, suspect or scene, can be analysed for chemicals such as dyes and cleaning products.
- Swab analysis can show body fluids, e.g. semen or saliva, that can be matched to the assailant or other substances, e.g. lubricants or gunpowder residue.
- Blood samples are used for the detection of drugs and/or alcohol. This is particularly important for suspects detained under the *Road Traffic Act 1988* (see Chapter 17) and in cases such as so-called 'date rape', where the victim is given a sedative like Rohypnol prior to being assaulted.
- Urine analysis can demonstrate the presence of alcohol, drugs and/or their metabolites much later than blood analysis, e.g. the metabolites of cannabis are detectable in the urine up to 46 days after ingestion.

Comparison Microscopy

- Objects, e.g. hair and fibres, retrieved from the victim or the crime scene can be compared under the microscope with those from the suspect to see if they match.
- Nail clippings can be matched to broken pieces of nail found at the scene by matching the nail striations.

PROBLEMS WITH TAKING SAMPLES
Informed Consent

Section 62 of *PACE 1984* allows the collection of intimate samples from a person in police custody but only with his consent. A detainee is not obliged to provide specimens for forensic examination or to undergo medical treatment or examination, except for intimate body searches (see later) but subsection 10 allows the court to make adverse inferences from a refusal to consent. Intimate samples must be taken by an HCP and require authorisation from an inspector or above, who must have 'reasonable grounds' to believe that the sample will prove or disprove the involvement of the suspect in a recordable offence. Police officers can take samples of head hair, nails, urine and saliva and perform external swabs, including mouth swabs. The detainee must be age of 17 or older in order to give a valid consent. If he is 14 to 17, then consent must be obtained from both the detainee and a parent or legal guardian. If he is younger than 14, then consent should be obtained from the parent or legal guardian only.

It may be very difficult to be certain that you have obtained informed consent, i.e. that the person fully understood the reasons for providing the samples and the possible future ramifications. This is particularly true for samples for blood alcohol and drug analysis as, by definition, the person is considered to be under the influence of drugs and/or alcohol. If in doubt, ensure that you have a witness to the fact that you have given the person a full explanation and make a full and detailed record of the conversation. If you doubt the capacity of the person to give consent through reason of mental illness or impairment (see Chapter 5), then either ask for a psychiatric assessment or take the samples in the presence of an 'appropriate adult' to help explain and oversee the procedure. **Never** take samples from an unconscious patient as this cannot be justified as being in the 'best interests' of the patient (see Chapter 5) except in **very exceptional circumstances** such as the comatose victim of a serious assault or an unconscious driver under the *Road Traffic Act 1988* (see Chapter 17) and even this is subject to debate. **Never** take samples by force if you cannot obtain consent.

Contamination

Locard's principle is 'Every contact leaves a trace'.

This means that trace evidence can be accidentally transferred from one object or person to another so you should **never** examine or take samples from both the parties involved in one incident. This is particularly true for cases that rely heavily on the forensic evidence for a conviction. In a murder case, the HCP who pronounced life extinct in the victim must never then examine the possible suspect. In a rape case, the suspect should never be examined at the same location as the victim by the same HCP or transported in the same vehicle.

CONTINUITY OF EVIDENCE
Taking Samples

The samples required depend on the type and nature of the crime committed and you should discuss this with the investigating officer prior to taking any samples but if in doubt, take the sample as there is unlikely to be another opportunity. Before commencing, check that the requesting officer has read out the correct part of the request for intimate samples as stated in *PACE 1984* and note that the Act requires that intimate samples may only be taken by a registered HCP. For blood samples obtained under the *Road Traffic Act 1988*, there is also a section that must be read out by the sergeant to both you and the detainee prior to the sample being taken (see Chapter 17).

Make sure you write that you have been provided with informed consent and take all the samples in the presence of the requesting officer. If you are taking blood, always swab the venepuncture site with an alcohol-free swab and use the forensic kits where available. You should label all your samples and place them in a tamper-evident bag, which is then labelled with the same details. Sign the bag then hand it to the requesting officer who will seal and also sign it.

Labelling

All samples and bags must be labelled in the order in which they were taken with the following:
- the name of the person providing the sample
- the hospital or custody number
- your initials, the date of birth of the person providing the sample, then the number of the sample, e.g. VGM/15021960/1—this is the exhibit number
- your name
- the place, date and time of the sample using the 24-hour clock.

Note that if more than one person is examined from the same enquiry, then item numbers should continue in series, even if they were taken on different days.

In Scotland, exhibits are known as productions.

Your Statement

Your statement should contain a numbered list of all the samples with the:
- exhibit number
- nature of sample

- site of the sample
- time of the sample, using the 24-hour clock
- seal number of bag.

For example:
'I took the following samples:
1. VGM/15021960/1—Dry swab taken from Mr. X's penile shaft at 18.05 hours. Seal No. B2543218
2. VGM/15021960/2—Wet swab taken from Mr. X's penile shaft at 18.06 hours. Seal No. B2543219'

Always give the name and rank of the police officer to whom you handed the samples and the time at which you did so, e.g. 'I handed the samples to DS Smith at 18.40 hours'.

See Table 4.1 and note the following:
- Blood taken for the purposes of the *Road Traffic Act 1988* must be drawn as a single sample of 8 mL, then divided equally into two 4 mL samples, preferably into the standard containers provided in the packs. In hospital, the single sample should be divided into two vials containing an anticoagulant such as fluoride and oxalate (see Chapter 17).
- Both urine and saliva can be collected by police officers. Urine should be collected in the vials provided, as these contain preservatives at the level suitable for alcohol analysis. Saliva and mouth washings can go into plain, sterile tubes.
- Only plain, sterile swabs should be used and they must not be placed in transport medium.
- Wet stains are sampled using a dry swab, but the swab should be moistened in distilled or tap water for dry stains. If tap water is used, then a control swab of the tap water should be provided. A further swab should be rubbed over the skin adjacent to the stain as a control sample.
- Note that many of the samples should be stored in a freezer so all containers must be shatter-proof.
- If instruments are required to collect samples, e.g. scissors or specula, then they must be sealed and disposable.
- Specula or proctoscopes can be moistened with sterile water but lubricants must never be used.
- Hair that appears to be contaminated, e.g. with semen, should be cut where possible or swabbed if the person objects. A control sample of hair should also be cut or swabbed.
- Pubic hair can be combed but never plucked.
- Nail clippings are preferable to scrapings, but the nails may be too short.

TABLE 4.1
Types of Samples and Methods of Their Processing

Sample Type	Reason for Analysis	Method of Sampling	Storage
Blood preserved (sodium fluoride and potassium oxalate)	Alcohol, drugs and volatile substances	8 mL venous blood	Refrigerate
Urine preserved	Alcohol and drugs	20 mL urine	Refrigerate
Saliva	Semen if oral penetration <72 hours ago	5–10 mL saliva	Freeze
Mouth swab	As for saliva DNA	Two sequential samples by rubbing swab around mouth	Freeze
Mouth washings	As for saliva	Rinse mouth with 10 mL sterile water and retain washings	Freeze
Skin swabs	Body fluids and other substances, e.g. lubricants	Dry swab for moist stains	Freeze
		Wet swab for dry stains	Freeze
Head hair	Body fluids, e.g. semen	Cut hair or swab area	Freeze
	Foreign particles or fibres	Remove visible items and use comb or tape	Freeze
	Control sample (suspect)	Cut 10–20 hairs close to scalp	Freeze
Pubic hair	Body fluids, e.g. semen	Cut hair or swab area	Freeze
	Foreign particles or fibres	Comb hair and collect debris	Freeze
Vulval swab	Body fluids if vaginal penetration <7 days or anal <3 days	Rub two sequential swabs over vulval area (moisten if required)	Freeze
	Lubricant if used or from condom <30 hours	Number in order taken	
Vaginal swab—low	As for vulval swab	Two sequential swabs under direct vision before speculum is passed Number in order taken	Freeze
Vaginal swab—high	As for vulval swab	Two sequential swabs using unlubricated speculum Number in order taken	Freeze
Endocervical swab	Only necessary if vaginal penetration <48 hours	One swab via the speculum	Freeze
Penile swab	Body fluids if intercourse <72 hours ago Lubricant if used or from condom <30 hours	Two sequential swabs from coronal sulcus and two from shaft and glans Number in order taken	Freeze
Perianal swab	As for penile swab	Two sequential moistened swabs from perianal area Number in order taken	Freeze
Rectal swab	As for perianal swab	Swab lower rectum after passing proctoscope 2–3 cm into anal canal	Freeze
Anal canal swab	As for perianal swab	Swab with proctoscope withdrawn	Freeze
Fingernails	Recovery of trace evidence	Cut or take scrapings with swab	Freeze

INTIMATE SEARCHES

Although not strictly related to the taking of forensic samples, a request to perform a nonconsensual intimate search on a detainee can cause the HCP concern so it is worthy of inclusion in this chapter.

Under Section 55 of *PACE 1984*, a 'registered doctor or nurse' can perform a nonconsensual intimate body search and the Act distinguishes between two groups of material for which such a search can be authorised. Section 55(a) deals with intent by a detainee to conceal dangerous weapons for use on either himself or others while in custody, while Section 55(b) deals with drugs. Intimate searches for drugs are limited to Class A drugs in Schedule 2 of the *Misuse of Drugs Act (MDA) 1971* (see Chapter 18) and these are usually heroin and cocaine. The inspector authorising the search must believe that the suspect has concealed drugs in a body orifice **and** that he intended to supply the drugs, which is an offence under Section 5(3) of the *MDA 1971*. This is known as 'appropriate criminal intent' in *PACE 1984*. An intimate body search excludes the mouth but involves the physical examination of the remainder of the orifices including the ears, nostrils, rectum and vagina so most HCPs are unwilling to perform it without consent. The defence organisations, the British Medical Association (BMA) and the General Medical Council (GMC) recommend that this be done under only very exceptional circumstances but there are two factors to consider before refusing:

1. Section 55 also allows for the search to be performed by a police officer of the same sex and the detainee may prefer that it be done by a doctor or nurse.
2. The risk posed to third parties by concealed weapons or drugs.

Note the HCP also has an obligation to warn the patient of the possible complications following the ingestion of certain drugs such as bowel obstruction and drug leakage leading to acute intoxication and possible death from overdose. The search for drugs can only be performed in suitable medical premises so it should never be done in a police station but the search for a concealed weapon may be done at either.

SUMMARY

This chapter gives the reader an overview of the history of DNA sampling, the different types of samples, both intimate and nonintimate, and sampling technique. It teaches the reader the correct methods of both taking and submitting samples and provides advice on the best way of completing the accompanying statement. It also warns the reader of the dangers of cross-contamination and taking nonconsensual samples, with a brief explanation of intimate searches.

CASE SCENARIOS

1. You have been asked to take intimate samples (penile swabs and pubic hair combing) from a 16-year-old boy, who has been accused of rape. Should you ask for the circumstances of the alleged assault and why?
2. Who needs to give consent to this procedure and who should be present during sampling? How can you be sure that it is informed consent?
3. You take the samples and hand them to the requesting officer, who asks you if you would be prepared to take samples from a second suspect, who is 14 years old. Should you agree?

See 'Answers to case scenarios'.

NOTE

1. *R v Kilkenny* (1991) 93 Cr. App. R. 287; [1992] 2 All ER 417.

USEFUL WEBSITES

Faculty of Forensic and Legal Medicine: www.fflm.ac.uk

CHAPTER 5

Consent

BOX 5.1
Necessity of Consent

'Every human being of adult years and sound mind has a right to determine what shall be done with his own body; and a surgeon who performs an operation without his patient's consent commits an assault, for which he is liable in damages', said Justice Cardozo in *Schloendorff v Society of New York Hospital, 1914*[1].

INTRODUCTION

Every person has the right to have his body integrity protected against invasion by others and only rarely can this be compromised, e.g. during arrest. Consent is the ethical precept that allows a patient to make invasion lawful—whether that invasion is into their body or their confidential information. Prior to 2003, there was no statutory definition of consent in UK law but Section 74 of the *Sexual Offences Act 2003* now defines consent as 'he agrees by choice and has the freedom and capacity to make that choice' (see Chapter 15). Case law (see Chapter 1) had already established that touching a patient without valid consent may constitute a civil or criminal offence as shown in Box 5.1.

TYPES OF CONSENT

Consent can be:
1. *Implied*—This is behavioural, e.g. a patient voluntarily undresses for examination.
2. *Express*—The patient gives permission orally or in writing.
   Note that both types of consent are equally valid although written consent does provide documentary

evidence, but it is the **reality** of consent that is important—a consent form signed in the absence of information is valueless. Note also that some procedures have a statutory requirement to obtain written consent and must not proceed without it, e.g. fertility treatment under the *Human Fertilisation and Embryology Act 1990*.

OBTAINING CONSENT

Consent is only valid if the following principles apply:
- The patient is legally competent and has capacity.
- The consent is voluntary and given freely without coercion.
- It is **informed**, i.e. the patient has been given **all** the information about the intention, nature and purpose of what is intended including the benefits and risks, possible side effects, any reasonable alternative treatments and the likely sequelae of refusing treatment.
- It is **appropriate**, e.g. consent to sterilisation does not include bilateral salpingectomy. Note that is only acceptable to perform additional procedures if it would not be safe to delay them, e.g. a life-saving manoeuvre. They should never be done purely for convenience.

Consent should be given to the clinician providing the treatment, as it is his responsibility but if he needs to delegate the task to another healthcare professional (HCP), he must ensure his delegate is adequately informed, qualified and trained for the task. Obtaining consent should also be a continuous process that starts well in advance of the proposed procedure, so the patient has ample opportunity to review his decision before the procedure starts.

The following information may be relevant when obtaining consent:

1. Details of the probable diagnosis and any further investigations necessary or desirable
2. The likely prognosis, with or without treatment
3. The options available for treatment, management or palliation with details of their possible benefits, risks and probabilities of success
4. The purpose and details of any proposed procedures, including side effects (see later)
5. Follow-up
6. The likely recovery time
7. A reminder that the patient has the option to change his mind at any time and that he has the right to a second opinion.

Remember to ALWAYS ask the patient if he has understood the information that he has been given and if he would like any more before he decides. Answer all questions as fully and honestly as possible and if you do not know the answer, say so.

DISCLOSURE OF RISK

The original landmark case regarding the duty of a doctor to warn patients of possible risks was that of *Bolam*[2] and it was based upon on whether the doctor had acted 'in accordance with a responsible body of medical opinion', which became known as the 'Bolam test'. In 1985 the case of *Sidaway v Board of Governors of the Bethlem Royal Hospital*[3] ruled that the decision about what degree of disclosure of risk was best calculated to assist a particular patient to make a rational decision was a purely clinical judgement—'doctor knows best'. Later cases meant clinicians had to disclose risks if they were **material**, i.e. a reasonable ('prudent') patient or doctor would attach significance to them, of a high incidence, of a low incidence but with potentially serious consequences or if a patient specifically asked, i.e. he attached significance to a particular risk. However, the doctor still did not have to disclose if he thought that it would be detrimental to the patient by invoking his 'therapeutic privilege'. This paternalistic approach ended in 2015, when the case of *Montgomery*[4] led to the ruling that a clinician must disclose **all** material risks **and** any to which it would be reasonable to consider that the patient may place significance. This means that you must talk to your patient and learn if he has any particular concerns. The information must also be provided in a way that the patient understands.

If the patient wishes to give consent without hearing all the information, he is entitled to do so but this **must** be recorded in the notes and he should be given opportunities in the future to change his mind if appropriate.

You must ALWAYS make a contemporaneous entry in the notes to state that consent has been obtained and write down what you told the patient—particularly a list of all the risks and complications.

ASSESSMENT OF CAPACITY

Capacity relates not to the final decision, but to the way in which the patient arrives at it and all adults are presumed to have capacity unless proved otherwise. Under the *Mental Capacity Act 2005* (see Chapter 16), a patient is deemed to have capacity if he can be shown to:

1. comprehend information that has been presented to him in a way that he can understand
2. retain that information long enough to make a particular decision
3. be able to weigh up that information
4. communicate that decision in a way that can be understood, which includes speech, hand gestures or blinking.

Patients should always be supported to make their own decisions wherever possible and they cannot be assumed to lack capacity if you do not agree with their decision, or it seems unwise. Note that capacity may fluctuate and that a patient may have the capacity to consent to simple procedures, but not to more complicated ones. Remember that refusal to consent requires a higher level of capacity than agreement and that patients who suffer from mental illness do not necessarily lack capacity.

It may be appropriate to ask a psychiatrist to see the patient, particularly if he is refusing potentially life-saving treatment. Assessment of capacity may be compromised by factors such as stress, pain, alcohol, drugs or coexisting illness, e.g. head injury but note that in law, alcohol intoxication alone does not make a person incapable of making decisions (see Chapter 17).

If you are in any doubt, ask for a second opinion.

LIMITS OF CONSENT

Criminal or unethical conduct cannot be made lawful just because a patient requests it. This includes:

• euthanasia
• maiming

- nontherapeutic sterilisation
- some cosmetic surgery
- experimental or unorthodox procedures.

CONSENT AND THE UNCONSCIOUS PATIENT

Clinical staff can treat unconscious patient in the absence of consent under the 'doctrine of necessity'. This means that as long as the clinician can justify his actions as being in the 'best interests' of the patient, he will be protected against any subsequent legal action. However, the treatment can only be justified if:

1. It saves life
2. And/or prevents further deterioration
3. And/or improves health
4. It is in accordance with established medical practice
5. The patient was competent and did not refuse treatment prior to losing consciousness.

The treatment must be limited to that required to satisfy these criteria if the patient is likely to regain capacity upon recovery. Proxy consent can be obtained if the patient has given authority through a Lasting Power of Attorney (LPA) under the *Mental Capacity Act 2005* or the *Adults with Incapacity (Scotland) Act 2000* (see Chapter 16) but **nobody else** can give consent on behalf of a previously competent patient.

In law, there are two standards adopted for making decisions on behalf of incompetent patients who have not previously appointed an advocate:

1. **'Best interests'** or **'objective'**—The decision-maker must choose the treatment that would be most beneficial to the patient. This standard is mainly used for those who have never been competent, but it is sometimes applied in emergency situations.
2. **'Substitutive judgement'** or **'subjective'**—The decision-maker must provide the treatment that the *patient* would have chosen had he still been competent. This standard is mainly used for those who were once competent but are no longer, e.g. *Airedale NHS Trust v Bland 1992/3*[5] where treatment was discontinued on the basis of being in the **'best interests'** of the patient (see Chapter 13). Substituted judgements tend to be based on quality, rather than quantity of life.

CONSENT AND IMPAIRED INTELLECTUAL ABILITY

Only a welfare attorney appointed under the *Mental Capacity Act 2005*, or the *Adults with Incapacity (Scotland) Act 2000* can give proxy consent if a patient over the age of 18 lacks capacity through impaired intellectual ability. Note that this proxy can act in all circumstances where the patient has been assessed as incompetent, but he cannot demand treatment that is judged to be against the patient's best interests. If no such 'decision-maker' has been appointed, treatment can only be given in the best interests of the patient and should preferably involve the guardian or relatives. Some cases should be referred to the Court of Protection (see Chapter 16) for guidance and/or authority, e.g. treatments that are not curative such as sterilisation, abortion or organ donation.

CONSENT AND THE MENTALLY ILL

See Chapter 16.

CONSENT AND MINORS

In England and Wales, the *Family Law Reform Act 1969* allowed minors of sound mind and aged 16 or over to give consent to surgical, medical or dental procedures. In Northern Ireland, the relevant Act was the *Age of Majority Act 1969* and in Scotland, it is the *Age of Legal Capacity (Scotland) Act 1991*. However, the case of *Gillick*[6] in 1985 led to the ruling that unless a statute or otherwise provides, a minor can give consent if they have sufficient understanding and intelligence to make the decision. This overrides the parental rights, but the judge recommended that the HCP should always try to obtain parental authority. This case also led to the 'Fraser Guidelines' but these specifically relate to sexual health and contraception.

The ruling was confirmed in the *Children Act 1989* and the *Children (Scotland) Act 1995*, which gave statutory power to mature minors younger than 16 years old to consent to treatment although the case of *Re R*[7] in 1992 modified the concept of the 'competent minor'. R was a disturbed girl of 15 who required sedation but refused medication during her lucid phases. The local authority applied for wardship to be able to administer treatment without consent and R appealed against it. The Court of Appeal ruled that the powers of the court were wider than parental since the court could override both consent and refusal of treatment and were not affected by the *Children Act 1989*. It also said that Gillick did not apply since maturity could not be assessed where the mental state fluctuated, so the order was upheld on the basis that R was not 'Gillick competent' and treatment could be authorised in her best interests. This meant that **refusal** to consent did not carry same weight as **agreement**. In England, Wales and Northern

Ireland, a court or a person with parental responsibility may authorise an investigation or treatment in the child's best interests if an apparently otherwise competent child refuses. In Scotland however, only the court can do this. As the numbers of competent children that have withheld consent to life-saving treatment have risen since the introduction of the *Children Act 1989*, there is now increasing recognition that such children do have a right to legal representation and that their views must be considered.

As with adults, all children aged 16 years or more should be assumed to have capacity unless proven otherwise and children under 16 should be assessed for capacity before deciding whether they can give informed consent. If the child is under 18 (16 in Scotland) and not competent, then a *competent* person with parental responsibility (see Chapter 14) can authorise investigations or treatments that are in the best interests of the child. Note that the authority of only one person is necessary for a therapeutic intervention, even if another refuses. If the intervention is nontherapeutic, e.g. male circumcision on religious grounds and two parties disagree, it is advisable to seek a court ruling. If that person refuses to give consent, then a clinician can still treat the child without consent if it is an emergency. If the treatment or investigation is nonurgent but still in the best interests of the child, then the clinician can ask either the local or the health authority to apply for a 'specific issue order' under the *Children Act 1989* (see Chapter 14). This allows the clinician to give the treatment without there being any other effects on the child's welfare, as may follow a wardship order. This is the most acceptable route to follow where the care of the child is otherwise good and the only point of disagreement is the withholding of consent, e.g. a child who requires a blood transfusion but whose parents are Jehovah's witnesses. It is probably more appropriate for the local authority to make the application, as they have a statutory responsibility to investigate and act in cases where the child may be at risk of appreciable harm and this would include the withholding of necessary treatment. Serious nontherapeutic interventions such as sterilisation should always be referred to the courts. Note that once a minor is made a ward of court, then no major treatment can be given without permission of the court (Fig. 5.1).

CONSENT IN SPECIAL CASES
Jehovah's Witnesses
An adult is entitled to refuse a transfusion, but he may be asked to sign a specific consent form to show that he understands the risks associated with not having a blood transfusion when it is clinically indicated. The clinician must also be satisfied that the patient is not under any pressure from his relatives to make his decision, i.e. there is no coercion. If the patient has made his wishes clear but then loses consciousness, it cannot be assumed that he would have changed his mind so a transfusion should still be withheld. The clinician must decide whether he is prepared to treat the patient under these circumstances and if not, then he is entitled to transfer the patient to the care of another clinician. Minors present a much greater problem. Under the *Children and Young Persons Act 1933*, it is a criminal offence to ill-treat, neglect or abandon a child younger than 16 years old so if a child dies, the result could be a charge of manslaughter. In the past, the solution used to be to make the child a ward of court, but now treatment is either instigated by the clinician, preferably a consultant, as being in the best interests of the child or given under a Specific Issue Order.

Prisoners
Prisoners cannot choose their doctor, but otherwise they have the same rights as anyone else and consent must be obtained before any treatment is given.

Intimate Samples
See Chapter 4.

Screening
Patients giving consent to screening tests should be aware of the following:
- The purpose of the test
- The likelihood of positive and negative findings
- The risks of false negative and positive results
- Any risks associated with the screening process
- Any medical, social or financial implications, e.g. preexisting medical conditions and travel insurance
- Follow-up.

Clinical Trials
The General Medical Council (GMC) produced guidance on consent to and good practice in research as part of their Good Medical Practice:
- Consent must be obtained on a special form that is tailored to the particular requirements of research and preferably by independent person.
- The research must be subject to an independent ethical review.
- The patient must be aware that participation is voluntary and that he can decline or withdraw at any time without any prejudice to his future care.

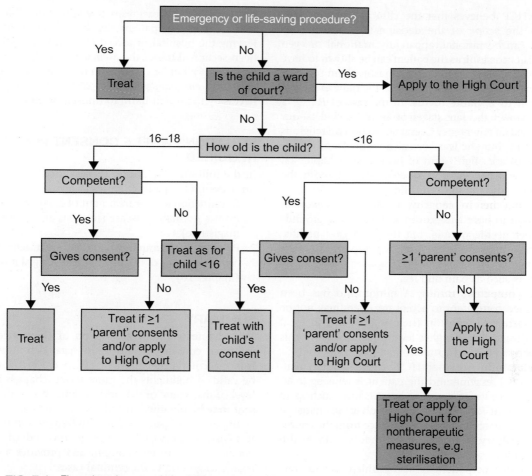

FIG. 5.1 Flow chart for consent in children—'parent' is anyone with parental responsibility.

- Patients without the capacity to consent should only be entered into trials where there is likely to be a therapeutic benefit and where similar research would not be feasible on competent patients.
- Children should only be entered into clinical trials with the consent of (preferably both) parents and the child if he is competent. If the parents disagree or refuse consent and it would be in the best interests of the child to be entered into the trial, then you should obtain legal advice.

Consent to Post Mortem and Removal of Human Tissue
See Chapter 11.

Consent and Dead Patients
The executors of the will can give consent on behalf of dead person, e.g. the release of records to an insurance company but it must be **all** the executors. If the person died intestate, then the descendants can apply for a 'letter of administration', but they must be the personal representatives of the deceased, which is not necessarily the next-of-kin.

Surgical Implants
Any device or prosthesis implanted surgically becomes the property of the person in whom it is implanted unless a special consent form is signed that gives rights of ownership to the Trust. After death, it forms part of the estate.

REFUSAL TO CONSENT
Competent adult patients have the right to refuse to consent to treatment, even when that refusal might result in harm or even death. This includes the instructions contained in valid Advance Decisions (see Chapter 13)

if the HCP believes that the clinical situation falls within the scope of the decision. The reasons for refusal can be rational, apparently irrational or even nonexistent as long as the patient can be shown to have capacity and he does not need to justify them.

There are very few exceptions to the right to refuse:

1. **Harm to a viable foetus**: In the case of *Re: S*[8], a woman in the late stages of an obstructed labour refused an emergency Caesarean section on religious grounds but she was overruled by the Family Division of the High Court of Justice (see Chapter 1), as it was necessary to save the lives of both the mother and the unborn child.
2. **Fluctuations in capacity**: In *Re MB*,[9] a woman refused to have a caesarean section on the grounds of her needle phobia, but the court gave permission to proceed on the basis that capacity to make particular decisions can be temporarily affected by factors such as pain and fear.
3. **The competent minor**: A minor who has been deemed competent to accept treatment may not be competent to refuse it. The case of *Re W*[10] in 1992 confirmed that a higher level of comprehension is needed to refuse treatment than to consent to it.
4. **Undue influence**: If an HCP believes that the treatment is lifesaving and the patient is refusing treatment because of coercion by a relative, such as in the case of *Re T*,[11] then the consultant in charge of the patient should ask for guidance from the courts.
5. **Compulsory treatment order** under mental health legislation (see Chapter 16).

A competent patient is also entitled to withdraw his consent at any time, even during a procedure and this wish must be respected. However, before stopping, the HCP should ascertain the problem, check that the patient's capacity has not changed and explain the consequences of abandoning the procedure. If stopping the procedure might endanger the life of the patient, then the HCP is entitled to continue until it is no longer the case.

Remember that if a patient refuses treatment and you are satisfied that he is competent and understands the consequences of his refusal, then you CANNOT assume that he would have changed his mind if he loses consciousness. You have no right to treat him under those circumstances and you could be successfully sued if he survives.

If the patient is judged to be incompetent, he can be treated in his best interests and restrained if necessary under the *Mental Capacity Act 2005* (see Chapter 16) in a manner that is proportionate to the degree of resistance and the least restrictive option possible. Note that a competent patient cannot be prevented from leaving the hospital or forced to return unless he has been sectioned under the *Mental Health Act 1983* (see Chapter 16), but he can be restrained under the *Criminal Justice and Immigration Act 2008* if this is deemed necessary to prevent harm to himself or others.

SITUATIONS WHERE CONSENT IS NOT REQUIRED

In the following situations, the examination can continue even if the patient refuses to give consent:

1. Examination and/or treatment of a patient suffering from a notifiable disease (requires an order from a magistrate)
2. Psychiatric examination and/or treatment under certain sections of the mental health legislation (see Chapter 16).

SUMMARY

This chapter explores all aspects of the concept of informed consent, including the legal definition and lists the criteria that must be satisfied for consent to be valid. It highlights the more recent changes in the level of disclosure of risk and explains how valid consent may be obtained in different circumstances, such as unconscious patients and children of varying age. It advises the reader how best to proceed when the patient refused to give consent and provides a useful legal background to the seminal cases.

CASE SCENARIOS

1. Alice is an unaccompanied 14-year-old girl who attends your clinic with symptoms of a urine infection, which you confirm by a dipstick urine test. She needs to be prescribed antibiotics, but she does not want her parents to be informed that she is there. What should you do?
2. You decide that Alice has the capacity to consent, and you give her the antibiotics. She returns a month later, crying and again alone. She tells you that she has taken a cocktail of unspecified drugs and drunk nearly a bottle of whisky. Her level of consciousness is depressed but she is adamant that she does not want any treatment and 'just wants to die'. What should you do now?

See 'Answers to case scenarios'.

NOTES

1. *Schloendorff v Society of New York Hospital* 105 NE 92 (NY, 1914).
2. *Bolam v Friern Hospital Management Committee* [1957] 1 WLR 583.
3. *Sidaway v Board of Governors of the Bethlem Royal Hospital* [1985] AC 871.
4. *Montgomery v Lanarkshire Health Board* [2015] SC 11 [2015] 1 AC 1430.
5. *Airedale NHS Trust v Bland* [1993] AC 789.
6. *Gillick v West Norfolk & Wisbech AHA* [1986] AC 112.
7. *Re R (A minor) (Wardship: consent to treatment)* [1992] Fam 11.
8. *Re S (Adult: Refusal of medical treatment)* [1992] 4 All ER 671.
9. *Re MB (Caesarean Section)* [1997] EWCA Civ 1361.
10. *Re W (A minor) (Medical treatment)* [1992] 4 All ER 627.
11. *Re T (Adult: Refusal of treatment)* [1993] Fam 95.

FURTHER READING

Decision making and consent. GMC; 2020.
Decision making and mental capacity. *NICE Guideline 2018,*
Good Medical Practice. GMC; 2013.
Reference Guide to Consent for Examination or Treatment. London: Department of Health; 2009.
Consent Tool Kit. BMA Publications; 2019.

USEFUL WEBSITES

General Medical Council: www.gmc-uk.org
Mind: www.mind.org.uk/information-support/legal-rights/consent-to-treatment/about-consent/
British Medical Association: www.bma.org.uk
NHS: www.nhs.uk/conditions/consent-to-treatment

CHAPTER 6

Confidentiality and Disclosure

INTRODUCTION

Confidentiality is an agreement that gives the confider not only the right to expect discretion and the confidant the right to hear the truth but also the obligation to ensure guardianship of the information received. Until 2000, the duty of confidentiality in the UK was solely an implied form of contract between the healthcare professional (HCP) and the patient, so unauthorised disclosure of professional secrets constituted merely a breach of contract and was only subject to civil proceedings. However, Article 8 of the *Human Rights Act 1998* states that 'Everyone has the right to respect for his private & family life, his home & his correspondence', so when the Act came into operation in October 2000, confidentiality became a statutory obligation. This change in status should not matter in practice, as confidentiality has always been an important part of the HCP–patient relationship and even forms part of the doctor's Hippocratic oath as shown in Box 6.1.

BOX 6.1
Hippocratic Oath

'Whatever things seen or heard in the course of medical practice ought not to be spoken of, I will not, save for weighty reasons, divulge'.

GENERAL DATA PROTECTION REGULATION

The *GDPR (General Data Protection Regulation) 2016* came into effect in 2018, replacing and modernising the *Data Protection Act 1998*. It outlines the roles and legal obligations of both data controllers (determine the means and purposes of processing data) and data processors (responsible for processing the data on behalf of the Controller). Article 4(1) of the GDPR defines personal data as 'any information relating to an identified or identifiable natural person ("data subject")' who can be identified either directly or indirectly by reference to an identifier such as a name or address'. Article 9 further defines 'special categories of data', which include race, religion, criminal convictions and health data.

The GDPR sets out six principles for data protection:
1. Processing must be lawful, fair and transparent. One of the main differences between the GDPR and the *Data Protection Act 1998* is that data are only held lawfully if the data subject has given express informed consent (see Chapter 5), which must be recorded, specific and can be withdrawn at any time.
2. The purpose must be limited to that which is 'specific, explicit and legitimate'.
3. The data held must be the minimum necessary for the stated purpose.
4. Data must be accurate and kept up to date.
5. The data should only be kept for the least amount of time possible with a time frame where feasible.
6. It must be held securely with safeguards against attacks and data breaches.

The GDPR also confers the following rights to the data subjects:
1. Right of access to their data and to amend it where necessary.
2. Right to erasure (right to be forgotten).
3. Right to object to their data being lawfully processed unless the data controller has legitimate grounds for overriding their request.

The Information Commissioners Office (ICO) replaced the Data Protection Registrar and registration has been replaced by notification. The Commissioner maintains a public register of data controllers and a general description of the type of processing performed by each data controller. Notifications are renewable annually.

The GDPR applies to all companies that process personal data about living people, but HCPs are subject to a further policy for handling and processing data—the Caldicott Principles.

CALDICOTT PRINCIPLES

The *Caldicott Report 1997* identified and examined 86 different dataflows of patient-identifiable information. It made 16 recommendations about the use of data within the health service, including:

1. Appointment of a Caldicott guardian within each Trust to oversee issues of confidentiality (usually the Medical Director).
2. Establishment of a programme to reinforce staff awareness of confidentiality and information security in the NHS.
3. Introduction of a new NHS number to replace other identifiers.
4. Introduction of standards and protocols against which to judge the justifications for information use.

It also listed the six Caldicott Principles, although a seventh was added following a revision of the Caldicott Report in 2013 and the eighth was announced in December 2020:

1. Justify the purpose(s) for using confidential information.
2. Only use confidential personal information if absolutely necessary.
3. Only use the minimum confidential personal information necessary.
4. Access should be strictly need-to-know basis only.
5. Everyone with access to confidential personal information should be aware of their responsibilities.
6. Comply with the law.
7. The duty to share confidential personal information is as important as the duty to protect patient confidentiality.
8. Inform patients and service users of how their personal information is used.

The principles of confidentiality and disclosure are set out for doctors in *Confidentiality: Good practice in handling patient information*[1] from the General Medical Council (GMC), in *The Code*[2] produced by the Nursing & Midwifery Council (NMC) for registered nurses and the standards set by the Health & Care Professions Council (HCPC) for registered paramedics. They are all closely aligned with the Caldicott Principles:

- Use the minimum amount of personal information and anonymise it where possible.
- Manage and protect the information correctly—those responsible for confidential information must ensure that it is adequately protected from improper disclosure, access or loss during storage, transfer and disposal. This includes information stored, sent or received by fax, computer and e-mail.
- Be aware of your responsibilities—clinicians and those working in professions with access to medical data like receptionists and social workers have a duty to refrain from disclosing information learned directly or indirectly in their professional capacity. Care must be taken when either discussing or talking to patients in public areas such as at the reception desk or on the telephone to avoid being overheard by third parties.
- Understand and comply with the law.
- Share relevant information for direct care with other HCPs, **unless** the patient has specifically objected to this. If a competent patient makes an informed decision that his information cannot be shared with other HCPs, it should be respected, even if it puts him at a therapeutic disadvantage. Note that information should not be circulated to others simply because they are HCPs and managers, and administrators should not have routine access to identifiable data. Note also that a clinician who is the subject of a complaint is prohibited from seeing the notes made by a colleague involved in the subsequent care of the patient concerned unless the patient gives consent for him to do so.

  Note that it is the responsibility of the clinician divulging the information to ensure that other HCPs are aware that it is confidential in nature
- Ask for explicit consent to share personal information for purposes other than direct care or local audit **unless** the disclosure is in the public interest or required by law (see 'Exceptions to the Rules of Confidentiality'). You must ensure that the patient is aware of the consequences, i.e. what will be disclosed and to whom, the reasons for any such disclosure and the likely sequelae.
- Tell the patient about any disclosures that he may not expect unless it would undermine the purpose or not be appropriate, such as disclosures in the public interest. Make a record of any disclosures you make and any that you decide not to with your reasoning for each.

- Keep your patients informed about their rights regarding their personal information and support their choices.

EXCEPTIONS TO THE RULES OF CONFIDENTIALITY
The Patient Gives Consent
Discussed earlier.

Disclosure in the Patient's Best Interests
Information necessary to allow emergency treatment of a patient may be disclosed without consent unless the patient has previously forbidden this while acknowledging the risks to himself. If a patient lacks the capacity to consent (see Chapter 5), then information may be disclosed in a nonemergency situation with the following provisos:
- It must be necessary for the ongoing care of the patient.
- The patient's dignity and privacy must be respected.
- The patient must be supported in being involved in all decisions about any disclosure.

You must also consider:
- If the lack of capacity could be temporary, and if it is, then the disclosure can be delayed until after their capacity has been restored.
- Whether the patient had expressed any preferences about the disclosure before they lost capacity and this should involve asking others such as their welfare attorney, independent mental health advocate, relatives or carers.

Note that you **must** share relevant information with anyone appointed to make health and welfare decisions on behalf of someone who lacks capacity (see Chapter 16).

If a person who lacks capacity asks you **not** to disclose information, then you must try to persuade them to agree, but ultimately, if you consider that sharing the information would be in their best interests, then you must do so.

Some nonconsensual disclosures may be done for more than one reason, e.g. a young child suspected of having suffered a nonaccidental injury, where disclosure would be justified both in the child's interest and in the public interest in the prevention of child abuse. NHS staff also have a statutory duty under the *Children Act 1989* to cooperate with a social services investigation and this includes disclosure of any relevant information (see Chapter 14).

Disclosure in the Public Interest
Public interest in the confidentiality of medical information may sometimes be outweighed by the public interest in disclosure to protect an individual or society from serious harm, e.g. terrorism or a potentially fatal communicable disease, but if so, it must be limited to the proper authorities or to those who may be at grave risk without the information.

When considering disclosure in the public interest, the HCP should consider the points raised in Box 6.2.

Record your reason(s) for disclosing the information in the notes, the steps that you have taken to gain consent (where safe and/or practical to do so) and take advice from your Caldicott Guardian if possible. In the UK, HCPs who disclose in the public interest must be prepared to justify their actions to their disciplinary bodies. In America, an HCP may be held as being negligent if he does **not** break confidentiality when made aware that his patient poses a serious danger to another person. In a case heard in 1976,[3] the judge ruled that a therapist had an obligation to use reasonable care to protect the intended victim—to warn them or others close to them, notify the police or take whatever other steps necessary. In 1997, changes to the *Ontario Medicine Act* made it mandatory for doctors to inform the authorities when a patient threatens serious harm to others and the doctor believes that violence is likely. In the UK, disclosure in the public interest remains an ethical rather than a legal duty and courts are wary of claims to justify a breach of confidentiality.[4] HCPs ought to be assured of the support of their professional bodies and there is also some protection in law. The

---

BOX 6.2
Disclosure in the Public Interest—Things to Consider

- Balance the benefits of disclosure against the potential harm.
- Assess the urgency of the situation.
- Exclude all other means of achieving the objective.
- Consider whether or not the subject might be persuaded to give consent or if this might make the situation worse.
- Inform the subject *unless* this might increase the risk of harm.
- Limit the disclosure to only that which is strictly necessary.
- Seek assurances that the information will only be used for the purpose for which it was intended.
- Be able to justify the decision.

> **BOX 6.3**
> **Reasons to Justify Disclosure to the Police**
>
> - The risk is real, immediate and serious.
> - The risk will be substantially reduced by disclosure.
> - Disclosure is the only means by which the risk can be minimised.
> - The disclosure is limited to that reasonably necessary to minimise risk.
> - The consequent damage to the public interest in confidentiality is outweighed by the interest in minimising risk.

Public Interest Disclosure Act 1998 provides protection for individuals who make certain disclosures of information in the public interest and allows them to bring action in respect of victimisation ('whistle-blowers').

If the police demand access to a patient's notes or enquire about attendance at the emergency department, the person in charge must not release the information unless they have consent from the patient or a court order. However, it should be noted that it is a criminal offence under Section 51 of the *Police Act 1964* to give misleading information, as this amounts to obstruction. A senior doctor may make an exception in cases where a serious crime has been committed, the application for release of information is made in writing by a senior police officer and where the following advice from a case heard in England in 1990[5] can be applied. These reasons are summarised in Box 6.3.

If a patient assaults an HCP, he can inform the police even if it means telling them that the patient has been seeking medical treatment, but the information must not contain any clinical details.

Disclosure to the Driver and Vehicle Licensing Authority (DVLA)

See Chapter 17.

Disclosure Under the *General Data Protection Regulation (GDPR) 2016*

Patients with capacity, including competent children younger than 18 years, or an authorised third party such as a solicitor can request access to their health records through a subject access request (SAR), which can be electronic, verbal or written and they do not need to give a reason. Parents with parental responsibility (see Chapter 14) can access their children's records if it is not deemed to be against the wishes of a competent child or not in the child's best interests. If the patient lacks capacity, access to their health records can be granted on the grounds of being in their best interests or with the authority of a nominated individual, such as welfare attorney.

A health record is defined as information relating to the patient made by or on behalf of an HCP, including doctors, dentists, nurses, pharmacists, paramedics, chiropodists, physiotherapists and other practitioners. It includes **all** medical notes including medical illustrations, videos, tape recordings, photographs, X-rays, computer files, genetic registers, disease-management registers, third-party medical reports, manual records, post-mortem reports and laboratory results. The minimum retention period is 10 years for personal health records and 25 years for maternity and obstetric records, but the Department of Health recommends that any medical record, or summary of it, should be retained for as long as it remains relevant to the long-term care of the patient.

Release to a third party can only be given with the written consent of the patient and it must state the nature and extent of the disclosure requested. Copies should be sent, not the original records.

The individual must be provided with a copy of their records within 28 days, unless additional information is sought, in which case, the 28 days starts from the receipt of that information. The time limit can be extended to up to 2 months if there are complex or numerous requests, but the individual must be informed of any likely delays within 28 days of the SAR. Patients are entitled to be given all the personal information held about them by the data controller but may be satisfied with only limited content depending upon the reason for the SAR. When provided with a copy of their health record, the patient is entitled to an explanation of any medical terms and should be informed of:

- The purposes of the data processing, e.g. delivery of healthcare, research or audit.
- The categories of personal data.
- The organisations with which the data have been shared.
- Their rights to amend inaccurate data or object to certain data.
- Whether any automated decision-making processes were used.
- Their right to complain to the ICO.

Initial access must be provided free of charge unless it is deemed 'excessive' or 'manifestly unfounded' by the ICO and information is exempt from disclosure if:

- It could cause serious physical or mental harm to the patient or a third party.

- It relates to a third party who has not given consent to disclosure, unless that person is an HCP who was involved in their care.
- It has been requested by a third party and the patient has specifically requested that some or all of the information is kept confidential, or it is subject to legal privilege.
- It is restricted by a court order.
- It relates to the storage or use of gametes, or an individual born via IVF.
- Disclosure is prohibited by law, e.g. adoption records.

It is a criminal offence under the *Data Protection Act 1998* to delete or amend health records in response to an SAR, but patients can apply to the ICO to have inaccurate records corrected or deleted.

Disclosure Under the *Access to Health Records Act 1990* and the *Access to Health Records (Northern Ireland) Order 1993*

The GDPR does not apply to deceased persons but the duty placed on HCPs to respect confidentiality extends beyond death, so although much of the *Access to Health Records Act 1990* and the *Access to Health Records (Northern Ireland) Order 1993* have now been repealed, the sections dealing with access to manual records relating to the deceased have been retained. Only the personal representatives of the deceased and anyone who may have a claim arising as a result of the patient's death can access the notes, but whereas the personal representatives are entitled to receive copies of all the notes, those with a potential claim can only access the parts of the notes relevant to the claim. Access can be denied for the same reasons as those given above for an SAR, but also if the record-holder believes that the patient gave the information on the basis that it would not be disclosed to the applicant and patients can request that a note be put in the records to that effect.

Disclosure to Employers and Insurance Companies

Where assessments are performed on behalf of a third party such as a pre-employment medical, the HCP has an obligation to release the results to the requesting employer and this may necessitate the disclosure of personal information. The potential employee must be informed of this and the possible consequences when his consent is sought for the examination. It is generally advisable to keep evidence of the patient's consent on their file. If the patient refuses to give consent, the assessment should not be done and the refusal documented. The *Access to Medical Reports Act 1988*

came into force on 1 November 1989 and applies to England, Wales and Scotland. There are separate regulations for Northern Ireland called the *Access to Personal Files and Medical Reports (NI) Order 1991*. These Acts give a patient the right of access to any medical report prepared for insurance or employment purposes by a practitioner who *is or has been responsible for his care*, so this **only applies to reports prepared by the patient's own GP**, not occupational health clinicians. The Acts also allow the patient to withhold consent, request amendments or stop the report. The patient can be refused access if the practitioner believes that the report might endanger his physical or mental health or that disclosure would reveal information about another identifiable person other than an HCP.

Confidentiality Within the Family

- **Minors:** Minors may wish to conceal their medical history from their parents and if they are 'Gillick-competent' (see Chapter 5), they have a right to confidentiality. The HCP still has an obligation to try to persuade the minor to inform his parents.
- **Spouses:** Spouses have no automatic right to information and this includes termination of pregnancy and sterilisation. Also, the HCP cannot contact the police in cases of marital violence without the consent of the patient, however frustrating that may be.

Disclosure for Teaching, Audit and Research Purposes

Clinical audit should ideally be carried out by HCPs with clear professional obligations to maintain confidentiality, but increasingly trusts and GP surgeries are commissioning third parties to carry out audits on their behalf. Commissioners of such services must ensure that their employees have firm contractual obligations regarding the preservation of confidentiality. The British Medical Association guidelines state that the disclosure of 'truly anonymous data' for teaching, audit, research or commercial purposes does not breach confidentiality. In the past, discussion about the use of anonymised information has focused on what can be considered to be truly anonymous, e.g. information such as date of birth, diagnosis or postcode may not identify an individual in isolation but can in combination. The use of minimal data identifying the patient's electoral ward, sex and year of birth is usually acceptable for administrative or research purposes, but if the patient cannot be adequately anonymised, consent should be sought. If it cannot be obtained, the information cannot be used for teaching or audit but if it is for research purposes, the ethics committee must decide whether the potential public benefit of the research outweighs the rights of the individual.

Adverse Drug Reactions

HCPs have both ethical and legal responsibilities to report suspected side effects or adverse incidents relating to drugs and medical devices to the Medicines and Healthcare products Regulatory Agency (MHRA) using the 'Yellow Card' system (see Chapter 18). To comply with the GDPR and the GMC guidelines on confidentiality, HCPs must only provide the patient's initials, age, gender and a local identification number or code, e.g. a hospital number. This information can still be used to cross-reference all reports and prevent duplication but there is no longer any need to get the consent of the patient.

Complaints

When investigating a complaint, reasonable efforts must always be made to obtain consent before identifiable health information is used, unless a delay would pose a risk to others. If the patient refuses to give consent, their views should be respected unless the public interest in protecting other people outweighs them. The GMC and NMC have powers to require the production of medical records for their investigation of complaints as part of the performance procedures involving doctors and nurses (see Chapter 10).

Genetic Information

Genetic information is bound by the same principles of confidentiality as any other, but there is an added dimension in that the information may have direct relevance to other family members. This can result in a conflict for the HCP between a duty of confidentiality to the patient and a duty to protect others from avoidable harm and suffering. The HCP should advise the patient about the implications of the test results and encourage him to share the information with his

---

> ### BOX 6.4
> ### Reasons to Consider Breaking Confidentiality Over Release of Genetic Information
>
> 1. The severity of the disorder.
> 2. The level of predictability of the information provided by testing.
> 3. What, if any, action the relatives could take to protect themselves or to make informed reproductive decisions, if they were told of the risk.
> 4. The level of harm or benefit of giving and withholding the information.[6]

---

relatives. If he refuses to do so, the HCP should consider the list shown in Box 6.4.

If the HCP believes that he must inform the relatives, this should be discussed with the patient and the reasons given. Wherever possible, the patient should not be identified to the relatives and if they do not wish to be told the information, it should not be forced upon them.

Disclosure to Tax Authorities

HCPs in private practice may disclose confidential information to the Tax Inspector, but every effort must be made to separate financial information from clinical records.

Disclosure to a Solicitor

Information regarding a patient can be released to his own solicitor but only with the patient's explicit consent and the notes must not relate to any other person.

Disclosure of Documents for Civil Litigation

Records are usually made available for litigation purposes through an SAR, but in medical negligence and personal injury cases, an application for disclosure can be made under Sections 33 and 34 of the *Senior Courts Act 1981*. These allow disclosure to the applicant and his legal or medical advisers prior to full disclosure (the point where all parties must produce all documents in their possession relevant to an issue in the litigation), although inspection may be limited to the latter two only. The patient's consent is necessary and 'relevant documents' include case notes, X-rays, laboratory reports and letters, but not reports prepared specially for the litigation. The record-holders do not need to obtain the consent of the patient, or any HCPs involved, but they should be informed, allowing them the opportunity to apply to the court and have it set aside if they so desire and circumstances permit. Section 35 of the Act gives the court the power to refuse to order disclosure if it would be injurious to the public interest. The courts may also order that an action be stayed where a patient making a claim of negligence refuses to allow access to relevant medical records.

Disclosure of Documents for Criminal Proceedings and Inquests

An HCP in the witness box has absolute privilege and is protected against any action for breach of confidence but he cannot refuse to answer questions on grounds of breach of confidentiality. In criminal proceedings, if an HCP refuses to disclose health records, the person seeking the information may apply to the court for a witness summons to be issued requiring the HCP to produce the information. This is covered by the rules on third-party disclosure, introduced in the *Criminal Procedure (Scotland) Act 1995* and the *Criminal Procedure & Investigations Act 1996*. The applicant must state specifically what information he requires, why it is material to the case and why he believes it is held by the third party. He must also give reasons why the HCP will not release the information voluntarily. The HCP (not the patient) then has 7 days to notify the court that he wishes to make representations, either in writing or at a hearing. If a hearing is requested, the HCP (or his representative) can bring up the issue of confidentiality or argue that the information requested is not material to the case. If, despite this, the witness summons is issued, the HCP must then provide the records or be found in contempt of court.

Police investigating a relevant or indictable offence (basically any offence where the penalty is a minimum of 5 years imprisonment) can obtain a search warrant from a magistrate under the *Police & Criminal Evidence Act (PACE) 1984*, but Section 11 of the Act excludes medical records and specifically excludes samples from the search. If the police want access to these, they must apply for a special order under Section 9 of *PACE* and this can only be issued by a judge. Such orders are rarely given and under very limited circumstances, e.g. stolen medical records. The HCP or health authority must be informed that the application has been made and they are given the opportunity to be heard by the judge before the order is issued. The only exception to this rule is in cases where the police are investigating acts of terrorism and an order may be given without such notice under Section 38B of the *Terrorism Act 2000*. Where possible, it is more appropriate that the records are presented as oral evidence by the clinicians that made them, as the issues involved are often very complex and judges are rarely medically qualified.

Some coroners or procurator fiscals have both medical and legal qualifications, but if a coroner wishes to see the medical notes, he must also apply for a High Court order, although HCPs will usually take them to the inquest on request. Similarly, most coroners will allow the Consultant in charge of the patient to see the post-mortem report before the inquest, although this practice has been criticised and it has been suggested that the Consultant might change the way in which he presents his evidence once given the benefit of hindsight. However, it should be borne in mind that the Consultant is entitled to attend the post mortem anyway—either as a hospital representative or where information has been sworn that he is responsible for the death.

STATUTORY DUTIES

There are some statutes that require the HCP to breach confidentiality, but only under very strictly controlled circumstances:

- The *Human Fertilisation & Embryology Act 1990* requires explicit consent for disclosure of information from a fertility clinic to the patient's GP and disclosure without consent that identifies the patient under other circumstances is a criminal offence.
- *Gender Recognition Act 2004*—it is an offence under Section 22 of this Act to disclose 'protected information' obtained in an official capacity. This information is defined as an application for gender recognition or the persons' gender history, although there are several exceptions to this rule.
- Notifications under the provisions of the *Factories Act and of the Control of Substances Hazardous to Health (COSHH) Regulations*. Employers are required to assess and control health risks arising from exposure to hazardous substances, including biological agents and body fluids and inform employees about them. Correspondingly, HCPs must declare their immune status so their employer can protect any vulnerable workers by removing them from exposure to a quantified risk. Currently, all HCPs who undertake duties that may expose them to the risk of contracting hepatitis B must provide evidence of immunity before starting work.
- Abortions must be notified to the Chief Medical Officer under the *Abortion Act 1991*.
- Known or suspected drug addicts must be notified to the Home Office under the provisions of the *Misuse of Drugs Act 1971* and *Misuse of Drugs (Notification & Supply to Addicts) Regulations 1985*.
- Births and deaths must be notified under the *NHS (Notification of Births & Deaths) Regulations 1982*. Note that birth and death certificates are public documents and copies can be obtained for a fee.
- HCPs must report known cases of female genital mutilation to the police under the *Female Genital Mutilation Act 2003*.
- Note that doctors are not under any statutory duty to report a death to the coroner, but they must complete the death certificate in such a way that any need for referral is made clear to the Registrar of Births and Deaths, who is under such a duty. If they do not, they can be accused of obstructing the coroner. If a doctor gives a false cause of death, he can be charged under the *Perjury Act 1911* and the *Births & Deaths Registration Act 1953*. It is also illegal to omit conditions that

TABLE 6.1 Notifiable Diseases 1981	
Acute encephalitis	Acute meningitis
Cholera	Diphtheria
Dysentery	Food poisoning (suspected and confirmed)
Infective jaundice	Lassa fever
Leprosy	Leptospirosis
Malaria	Marburg disease
Measles	Ophthalmia neonatorum
Paratyphoid fever	Plague
Rabies	Relapsing fever
Scarlet fever	Small pox
Tetanus	Tuberculosis
Typhoid fever	Typhus fever
Viral haemorrhagic fever	Yellow fever
Whooping cough	Ebola

may have contributed to the death, even if it may cause distress to the relatives.

- Certain infectious diseases must be notified to the local authority under the *Public Health (Infectious Diseases) Regulations 1988*, *Public Health (Control of Disease) Act 1984* and the *Health Protection (Notification) Regulations 2010* (Table 6.1).
- Any person with information that might prevent an act of terrorism must inform the police (and/or the armed forces in Northern Ireland) under the *Prevention of Terrorism (Temporary Provisions) Act 2000*.
- There is a statutory duty under Section 72 of the *Road Traffic Act 1988* to give information that may identify a driver who is suspected of having committed a road traffic offence, but staff should only release the name and address, not any medical information.

REMEDIES FOR BREACH OF CONFIDENTIALITY

A patient can claim damages for improper disclosure of information about his health even if he did not suffer financially, and it can also be the basis of a complaint to the Health Service Commissioner. Breach of confidentiality is not defamation or slander as the information disclosed is usually true—the fault lies in the inappropriate disclosure. For a breach of confidentiality to be said to have occurred:

1. The information divulged must be confidential
2. It must have been divulged in confidence
3. There must be unauthorised use of information to the detriment of the person to whom it relates. Possible consequences for the HCP include:
1. **Disciplinary proceedings**—up to and including being struck off
2. **Civil proceedings**—where the HCP may have to pay compensation
3. **Criminal proceedings.**

SPECIALISED DOCTORS

1. **Prison Doctors**—Prisoners cannot choose their doctor but otherwise they have the same rights as free persons and consent to treatment must be given freely.
2. **Armed Forces Medical Officer (MO)**—No MO can be required to treat a patient in accordance with a given policy when it is not in the patient's best interests. However, service personnel must accept some loss of confidentiality, e.g. the MO might be required to discuss cases with his Commanding Officer (CO) in the interests of the unit as a whole, although these circumstances should be rare. The CO is obliged to respect the confidential nature and source of the information and the disclosure should be limited to the essential minimum. The individual should also be informed of the disclosure and the reasons why the MO considers it necessary. Informed consent to disclose voluntarily should be obtained wherever possible, and the MO would be advised to discuss the matter with his medical defence organisation.
3. **Expedition Doctors**—Similar to (2).
4. **Occupational Health Physicians and Nurses**—These are employees of the company, but they still have a duty of confidentiality. If they are required to perform medical examinations, then the nature of the examinations and the need for disclosure of any findings should be set out in the contract. They should only treat or refer patients with the cooperation of the GP unless in an emergency.
5. **Forensic Medical Examiners (FMEs), Custody Nurse Practitioners (CNPs) and Custody Paramedics**—It is often difficult to ensure confidentiality when examining detainees in custody, as the practitioner may need to be chaperoned by a police officer. It is important that the practitioner makes his role clear to the detainee and obtains consent,

especially when conducting an examination under Section 4 of the *Road Traffic Act 1988* where 'no part of the examination may be regarded as confidential' (see Chapter 17). Detainees are not obliged to submit to examination or treatment or to provide specimens and the practitioner must always obtain consent or risk being sued for assault.

SUMMARY

This chapter explains the concepts of the confidentiality of personal information and disclosure. It outlines the areas where disclosure is essential, appropriate and where it is not permitted. It expands on the two main policies for handling and processing data within the healthcare domain—the General Data Protection Regulation and the Caldicott Principles and provides detailed information on their application. It lists the statutory duties of disclosure for the HCP and covers the different obligations of clinicians who work in more specialised areas.

CASE SCENARIOS

1. Two police officers come to your clinic and ask for a summary of the medical record of a patient who attended for treatment of an injury earlier that day. Do you have to provide it? Do you need the consent of the patient? What information do you need to make an informed decision?
2. The police do not have any legal grounds to request the information and your patient declines consent to release of their medical notes, so you refuse to give the police officers the summary. They return the following week with a court order, do you now have to release the notes?
3. You have a patient called Jon, who has recently tested positive for HIV and you tell him that he must warn his partner Jane, who is also one of your patients. He tells you that he doesn't want to tell

her, as he is frightened that she would leave him and he is adamant that she is not at risk as they always use a condom—what should you tell him?
4. Jane attends the clinic a month later to inquire about starting the oral contraceptive pill, as she says that both she and Jon are 'fed up with condoms'. She does not seem aware of Jon's HIV status, so should you tell her?

See 'Answers to case scenarios'.

NOTES

1. General Medical Council. *Confidentiality: good practice in handling patient information.* London: GMC; 2017.
2. Nursing & Midwifery Council. *The Code: professional standards of practice and behaviour for nurses, midwives and nursing associates.* London: NMC; 2015.
3. *Tarasoff v Regents of the University of California* 529 P 2d 55 (Cal, 1974); 551 P 2d 334 (Cal, 1976).
4. *X v Y* [1988] All ER 648.
5. *W v Egdell* [1990] Ch 359; [1990] 1 All ER 835.
6. British Medical Association. *Human genetics: choice and responsibility.* Oxford: OUP; 1998.

FURTHER READING

Nursing & Midwifery Council. *The Code: professional standards of practice and behaviour for nurses, midwives and nursing associates.* London: NMC; 2015.
General Medical Council. *Confidentiality: good practice in handling patient information.* London: GMC; 2018.

USEFUL WEBSITES

www.ico.org.uk/for-organisations/uk-gdpr-guidance-and-resources/
www.homeoffice.gov.uk
General Medical Council: www.gmc-uk.org
Nursing & Midwifery Council: www.nmc.org.uk
HCPC: www.hcpc-uk.org
UK Caldicott Guardians Council (UKCGC): www.ukcgc.uk

Clinical Governance and Risk Management

WHAT IS CLINICAL GOVERNANCE?

When the NHS was established in 1948, there was no explicit consideration given to the quality of the healthcare it provided and it became apparent that the standard of care offered by the NHS varied greatly between hospitals, between departments in the same hospital and between general practices. In 1997, in the White Paper *New NHS Modern & Dependable*,[1] the government made it a statutory duty for all healthcare professionals (HCPs) to become involved in a quality agenda. This Paper set out a 10-year strategy for the NHS with a huge emphasis on quality and introduced the concept of corporate governance. It also promised to modernise the NHS, improve communication and make services quicker, more convenient and more consistent.

The National Institute for Clinical Excellence (NICE) was established in 1999, then joined with the Health Development Agency in 2005 to become the National Institute for Health and Clinical Excellence. In 2013, the *Health & Social Care Act 2012* renamed it as the National Institute for Health and Care Excellence

(but still abbreviated to NICE) to reflect its new role in social care. NICE is no longer part of the NHS, as it is now an executive nondepartmental public body of the Department of Health. It was established to end the so-called 'postcode lottery', where the decision whether patients received treatment depended upon the policies of whichever health authority they came under, but it is now best known for the development of high-quality evidence-based clinical guidelines and determinations of cost–benefit analyses for proposed innovative treatments. Its Scottish equivalent is Health Improvement Scotland (HIS), which was established by the *Public Services Reform (Scotland) Act 2010*.

There are three elements to the strategy for improving quality in the NHS:

1. **Set clear national quality standards**—through NICE or HIS
2. **Ensure local delivery of high-quality clinical services**—through clinical governance, Continued Professional Development (CPD—to ensure that HCP knowledge is contemporary) and professional self-regulation and revalidation (to monitor HCP performance)
3. **Monitor delivery of quality standards**—through the Care Quality Commission (CQC) (Fig. 7.1)

Clinical governance is central to the strategy and has been shown in Box 7.1. There are four key parts to clinical governance:

1. **Clear lines of responsibility and accountability for the overall quality of clinical care**—ultimately the Chief Executive of the Trust is responsible, but a designated senior clinician should ensure that systems for clinical governance are in place and that they are being monitored.

> **BOX 7.1**
> **Definition of Clinical Governance**
>
> 'A system through which NHS organisations are accountable for continuously improving the quality of their services and safeguarding high standards of care by creating an environment in which excellence in clinical care will flourish', said Scally and Donaldson.[2]

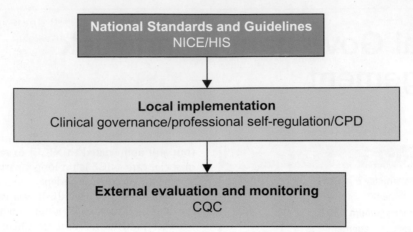

FIG. 7.1 Elements for improving quality in the NHS. *CPD*, Continued Professional Development; *CQC*, Care Quality Commission; *HIS*, Health Improvement Scotland; *NICE*, National Institute for Health and Care Excellence.

2. **A comprehensive programme of quality improvement activities**—these include clinical audit, participation in National Confidential Inquiries, implementation of NICE guidelines, staff training and CPD, safeguarding of information and record storage, research and development.
3. **Clear policies aimed at managing risk**.
4. **Procedures to identify and remedy poor performance**—these include incident reporting, complaints procedures, peer review and disciplinary procedures.

The Clinical Governance 'framework' refers to the infrastructure, processes and systems in place within an organisation in order to monitor and manage the quality of service provision, and thereby encompass, evidence and account for these key attributes. There are generally considered to be seven pillars to this framework:

1. Risk management
2. Clinical effectiveness
3. Patient, public and carer experience and involvement
4. Communication
5. Education and training
6. Staff management and training
7. Strategic capacity and capability.

The aim of clinical governance is to develop an open learning culture that shares information and makes changes that will improve the quality of care such that there are consistently better outcomes for the patients. This also involves primary care groups, including dentists, pharmacists, district nurses and opticians for whom their relative isolation can make this process very difficult. The Clinical Governance Support Team (CGST) trains and supports NHS organisations and their staff in the development of clinical governance systems. A crucial component is **risk management**, i.e. the ability to detect, analyse and learn from events such as adverse incidents (AIs) and systems failures.

WHAT IS RISK MANAGEMENT?

Risk management (RM) can be defined as a proactive approach which:

1. **Addresses** the various activities of an organisation
2. **Identifies** the risks that exist
3. **Assesses** those risks for potential frequency and severity
4. **Eliminates** the risks that can be eliminated
5. **Reduces** the effect of those that cannot be eliminated
6. **Establishes** financial mechanisms to absorb the financial consequence of the risks that remain.

The key aim of RM is to reduce the cost of risk.

PRINCIPLES OF RISK MANAGEMENT
Identification of Risk

In order to manage a potential risk, it must first be identified, i.e. what is the risk? How could it occur? What is the likely effect of the risk if it is not correctly managed? Examples of nonclinical risks would be physical hazards such as the storage of dangerous gases or working practices such as inadequate training on lifting patients. A clinical AI occurs when a patient is unintentionally harmed by medical treatment, e.g. drug errors, awareness while under anaesthetic and unexpected deaths or complications.

Analysis

Once the risk has been identified, it must then be analysed. The questions that must now be asked are: How often is the risk likely to occur? How much is it likely to cost—both to manage and if it is not controlled? What are the potential effects of both efforts to manage the risk and what could happen if the risk is ignored? There are many different methods of risk identification and analysis, including questionnaires, historical analysis, checklists and physical inspection.

Control

The next step is to consider the measures that must be taken in order to control the risk. It may be possible to totally eliminate the risk or at least avoid it, but it may only be feasible to make it either less likely or cheaper to deal with the outcomes. Examples of such measures include physical controls such as controlled drugs cupboards or restricted-access areas and others, e.g. training programmes on lifting or handling hazardous materials.

Funding

Funding for RM is part of every hospital budget, as detailed later.

WHY DO WE NEED RISK MANAGEMENT?
Altruism

The majority of HCPs feel a personal and professional responsibility to provide patients with the highest possible standard of care and expect to work in a safe environment in an industry with the same aims.

Legislation

Trusts must comply with legislation such as the *Health & Safety at Work Act 1974*, as failure to do so can result in fines, injunctions and the prosecution of individual managers.

Litigation

Both patients and staff are now far more inclined to take legal action and to seek compensation than in the past. Changes in the regulations on Legal Aid means that the entitlement of a minor to Legal Aid is no longer based on the parents' finances so there are more claims for birth injuries. Following the introduction of

Crown Indemnity in 1990, Trusts are also vicariously responsible for acts of negligence by their staff and must meet any resultant claims settlement and indirect expenses. HCPs are no longer obliged to be members of a defence organisation, although it is still recommended, as the cover does not extend to the medico-legal costs of inquests or referrals to disciplinary bodies such as the General Medical Council (GMC), Nursing and Midwifery Council (NMC) or (Health and Care Professions Council (HCPC).

Media Pressure

Incidents such as the Bristol Inquiry into the Paediatric Cardiac Surgical service and the Cleveland Inquiry where children were allegedly misdiagnosed as being sexually abused by their parents cause headline news and shake the public faith in HCPs. It is vital to show that there are systems in place for the early detection of any future problems and for a rapid response to any questions raised.

CNST AND CNSGP

The Clinical Negligence Scheme for Trusts (CNST) was implemented in April 1995. It was established under Section 21 of the *NHS & Community Care Act 1990*, although it is now regulated by Section 71 of the *NHS Act 2006*, as amended by the *Health & Social Care Act 2012*. It is administered by NHS Resolution and owned by its members who determine its policies and monitor the performance of the contracted managers. On 1 April 2013, independent sector providers of NHS care were allowed to join and cover was extended to include inquest costs.

Membership is voluntary but all NHS Trusts in England are members and it is basically a 'pay-as-you-go' insurance scheme against large negligence costs, i.e. only sufficient money is collected each year to pay out expected claims falling due that year. Excesses are used to offset contributions the following year or refunded to members, but the latter is rare. Cover is on 'claims paid' basis, i.e. the Trust must be a member at the time of the incident, the time that the claim is made and the time that the claim is settled and it includes defence legal costs. Cases arising before 1 April 1995 are dealt with by the Existing Liabilities Scheme (ELS), which is funded by the Department of Health and Social Care (DHSC) and managed by NHS Resolution.

Contributions are set according to the level of claims made against individual Trusts and they are adjusted for risk management and claims handling expertise, turnover and activity. This leads to the development of minimum objective standards of RM for each activity category of Trusts which, when achieved, allow the Trust to be considered for a contribution discount. This means that clinical incident reporting and the development of RM is no longer an optional extra for Trusts.

In April 2019, the Clinical Negligence Scheme for General Practice (CNSGP) and the Existing Liabilities Scheme for General Practice (ELSGP) were introduced. The CNSGP provides general practice staff with indemnity cover for claims relating to the provision of NHS primary medical services **from** 1 April 2019 onwards and the ELSGP provides cover for claims made prior to that date.

Note that the ELSGP **only** applies to healthcare staff who were members of either the Medical Protection Society (MPS) or Medical Defence Union of Scotland (MDDUS) at the time of the incident. Members of other Medical Defence organisations must speak to their indemnity provider directly.

CNSC

During the COVID-19 pandemic, the Clinical Negligence Scheme for Coronavirus (CNSC) was set up to meet any liabilities arising from the special healthcare arrangements established under the *Coronavirus Act 2020*, such as staff being directed to work in areas outside their normal expertise.

RM STANDARDS

There are three levels:
1. **Policy**—adequate documentation of effective risk management processes and systems.
2. **Practice**—implementation of the policies described in Level 1.
3. **Performance**—the Trust can show that it is monitoring its compliance with the policies and acting upon the findings.

NHS RESOLUTION

On 1 April 2017, NHS Resolution was formed to help the NHS to resolve claims fairly and quickly with an emphasis on sharing lessons learnt to improve clinical practice and reduce costs to preserve resources for patient care. There are four key service areas:
- Risk management in NHS Trusts and management of claims and litigation. In 2017/2018, only 1% of cases went to court with the majority being resolved through other methods such as mediation.
- Practitioner Performance Advice (PPA) (formerly known as the National Clinical Assessment Service (NCAS)), which provides impartial, expert advice to healthcare organisations with concerns about the performance of individual doctors, dentists or pharmacists.
- Primary Care Appeals (PCA) (formerly the Family Health Services Appeals Unit (FHSA)), which deals with the fair and prompt resolution of disputes between primary healthcare contractors and the commissioners of primary care services such as Clinical Commissioning Groups (CCG).
- Safety and learning—helping the NHS to understand and learn from disputes, complaints and claims.

NHS Resolution also manages two nonclinical schemes under the Risk Pooling Schemes for Trusts (RPST):
- Property Expenses Scheme (PES)—this covers 'first party' losses like theft or damage to property that occurred on or after 1 April 1999.
- Liabilities to Third Parties Scheme (LTPS)—this covers nonclinical claims, including employers and public liability.

FUNDING FOR CLAIMS IN WALES

NHS Trusts and Health Authorities in Wales can join the Welsh Risk Pool, which is part of the NHS Wales Shared Service Partnership (NWSSP) Legal and Risk Service and covers both clinical and nonclinical risks. The excess varies with each individual case and the premium paid by each Trust is a percentage of the Trust budget. The Pool has a similar set of RM standards to the CNST and the same emphasis on patient safety and outcomes.

The General Medical Practice Indemnity (GMPI) scheme for Wales was introduced in April 2019 to provide general practice staff with indemnity cover for claims related to the provision of NHS primary medical services **from** 1 April 2019 onwards. GMPI also operates the Existing Liabilities Scheme, which covers claims made prior to 1 April 2019.

FUNDING FOR CLAIMS IN SCOTLAND AND NORTHERN IRELAND

In Scotland, all NHS boards, special national boards and the Mental Welfare Commission for Scotland must be members of the Clinical Negligence and Other Risks

Indemnity Scheme (CNORIS), which covers both clinical and nonclinical claims. It is managed by National Services Scotland (NSS) and the Scottish Central Legal Office (CLO) acts for the Trusts. Trusts must pay for all claims costing less than the CNORIS deductibles threshold (currently £25,000) and the Scottish Government Health and Social Care Directorates (SGHSCD) funds all losses above that level.

In Northern Ireland, where the level of litigation is much higher, each health and social care trust must provide its own indemnity, funded by the Department of Health, Social Security and Public Safety. There are no RM standards and the Trusts get their legal advice from a list of approved solicitors.

There are no state-backed schemes for GPs that provide NHS services in Scotland or Northern Ireland and GPs in Northern Ireland often pay thousands of pounds for indemnity cover.

CLAIMS REPORTING

Both the CNST and the ELS rely upon their members reporting claims directly to them using the 'Claims Reporting Wizard'. This enters the information into a bespoke electronic Claims Management System (CMS) using codes that define:

- The date and location of the incident and the date on which it was reported to NHS Resolution
- The likely cause, based on the information provided
- The nature of the injury.
- The clinical specialty(ies) involved.

The CMS will also record the date of resolution of the claim, either through payment of damages or the successful defence of a nonmeritorious claim.

LIABILITIES

- In 2017/2018, NHS Resolution received 10,683 claims (including potential claims) under its clinical negligence schemes and 3570 nonclinical.[3]
- By 31 March 2017, NHS Resolution still had 29,420 'live' claims and CNST claims took an average of 1.65 years to settle from the date of notification to NHS Resolution to the date that compensation was agreed, or the case was discontinued by the claimant.
- The highest number of claims were related to surgery, but the highest cost was for obstetric cases.
- Note that an important type of liability is the IBNR ('incurred but not reported') liability, i.e. an incident has occurred that is likely to cost the Trust

or the CNST money, but it has either not yet been reported or paid.

INCIDENT REPORTING

The National Reporting and Learning System (NRLS) is a central database of patient safety incidents and the data are analysed to identify risks, hazards and opportunities to improve patient care. The NHS encourages both the general public and healthcare staff to report AIs to the NRLS, even if they do not result in any harm, as they help Trusts to learn from their mistakes, share that learning and improve patient care. The general public can report incidents directly via the e-form provided on the NHS England website, whereas healthcare staff must use their local risk management system, which then uploads the information onto the NRLS. Note that the NRLS cannot be used to investigate individual reports and is solely intended as a learning resource for Trusts. There are plans to replace it with the 'Learn from patient safety events (LFPSE) service', which should be easier to access, provide better data and will allow access from other care settings, such as primary care.

An AI is defined as 'an event that causes, or has the potential to cause, unexpected or unwanted effects that will involve the safety of patients, staff, users and other people'.[4] Most Trusts use one incident form for all AIs, regardless of origin, but some separate clinical incidents from nonclinical. Some allow staff to use other avenues such as speaking directly to their line manager or email and accept anonymous reporting. While the latter may be essential for incident reporting to be a blame-free process, it can make it very difficult to fully investigate an incident. Most Trusts also give their staff training in incident reporting—both in the actual process and what constitutes an AI, but there is little standardisation between Trusts over what is considered to be an AI. AIs are common and they are only rarely the result of a single failure in the process, such as one individual. The surgeon may be criticised when an operation goes wrong, but it may be that they were using inadequate equipment or had insufficient light. It has been shown that adverse conditions such as high workload, inadequate supervision or poor communication increase liability to error.[5] This means that investigations that consider only the acts of individual HCPs are inadequate and may be misleading. They also serve to discourage future reporting.

Incident data should be subjected to analysis, both at a local and a corporate aggregate basis, in order to reap the most benefit from it. It is particularly important to document near misses and to identify common themes in order to predict and prevent future incidents.

The effectiveness of incident reporting can be measured in three ways:

1. The number of changes in practice that have resulted from it.
2. Its success in alerting the Trust to potential complaints and/or litigation.
3. The amount of feedback given to clinicians.

In order for a reporting scheme to be effective it must:

- Be mandatory
- Be confidential
- Foster a blame-free culture of learning and enquiring to encourage reporting
- Provide information about general organisational failures as well as specific events
- Categorise serious adverse events and research them to identify trigger factors
- Have a system for analysing and disseminating information and lessons from incidents and near misses
- Implement the important lessons and make any necessary changes
- Provide support and feedback to the staff involved to give positive reinforcement.

CARE QUALITY COMMISSION (CQC)

The CQC was established in 2009 by the *Health & Social Care Act 2008* to be an independent regulator of health and social care in England. It replaced the Healthcare Commission, the Commission for Social Care Inspection and the Mental Health Act Commission, with the aim of providing a more integrated approach to the registration, monitoring, inspection and regulation of all categories of health and social care providers in England.

Any person (individual, partnership or organisation) who provides any regulated activity, as defined in the *Health & Social Care Act 2008*, must register with the CQC and in order to do so, they must prove that they are:

- safe
- effective
- caring
- responsive
- well-led.

Once they have tendered the extensive application form intended to show whether they meet the fundamental standards of the CQC, the care provider must submit to a thorough preregistration inspection prior to becoming registered with the CQC. They are then subject to a postregistration inspection, which is usually done without warning and leads to a rating:

- Outstanding—performing exceptionally well
- Good—performing well and meeting the standards
- Requires improvement—not performing as well as it should and must follow the instructions given by the CQC to address the concerns prior to the next inspection
- Inadequate—service is performing inadequately and subject to sanctions by the CQC.

Care providers are legally obliged to display their rating and adhere to the judgements and recommendations made by the CQC Inspectors. The CQC can take the following actions:

- Issue requirement or warning notices that set out what changes the care provider must make and by when
- Change the registration to limit what the provider can do
- Place the provider in special measures, which involves close supervision to help them improve
- Hold the provider accountable to their failings by issuing cautions, fines or even prosecution where people have been harmed or put at serious risk.

SUMMARY

This chapter gives an overview of the concepts of clinical governance and risk management within the NHS, primary care and the social care sector. It then goes into greater detail and explains what each entails, including standards, regional funding and why they are necessary for optimum patient care. It then discusses litigation, claims management and liabilities, and the importance of adverse incident reporting. It also provides a summary of the role of the Care Quality Commission.

NOTES

1. Department of Health. *The new NHS: modern, dependable.* London: HMSO; 1997.
2. Scally, G., Donaldson, L. Clinical governance and the drive for quality improvement in the new NHS in England. *BMJ.* 1998;317:1725–1727.
3. NHS Resolution. *Factsheet 3—Claims information. NHS;* 2017/2018.
4. Department of Health. *An organisation with a memory: report of an expert group on learning from adverse events in the NHS chaired by the Chief Medical Officer.* London: DH; 2000.
5. Vincent, C., Taylor-Adams, S., Stanhope, N. Framework for analysing risk and safety in clinical medicine. *BMJ.* 1998;316:1154–1157.

FURTHER READING

NHS Executive. *Clinical governance: quality in the new NHS.* Department of Health, 1999.

NHS Resolution. *Reporting claims to NHS Resolution, 2017.*

NHS Resolution (GPs). *Reporting guidelines—General Practice Indemnity, 2021.*

USEFUL WEBSITES

NICE: www.nice.org.uk

NHS Resolution: www.resolution.nhs.uk

NWSSP: www.nwssp.nhs.wales

CNORIS: www.clo.scot.nhs.uk

Reporting an adverse incident: www.england.nhs.uk/patient-safety/report-patient-safety-incident

Care Quality Commission: www.cqc.org.uk

CHAPTER 8

Handling Complaints

INTRODUCTION

On 1 April 2009, the new NHS and social care complaints procedure was introduced in England under the *Local Authority Social Services & NHS Complaints (England) Regulations 2009* and it applies to all 'responsible bodies', as defined in the regulations:

- NHS bodies and all other providers of NHS healthcare, including primary care and commissioning bodies.
- 'Independent providers', defined as independent sector and voluntary organisations that provide healthcare under an arrangement made with an NHS body.
- Local authority adult social services
Responsible bodies must:
- keep a record of all complaints
- record any lessons learnt
- analyse and monitor complaints as part of their clinical governance procedures
- provide an annual report.

The procedure is now a two-step process:

1. **Local resolution**—the complaint is investigated by the organisation being complained about and an attempt is made to resolve the complaints at a local level. If the complainant is not satisfied, they can apply for the complaint to be taken to the second stage.
2. **Parliamentary Health Service Ombudsman (PHSO)**—the PHSO performs an independent investigation of the complaint, both formally and informally, if local resolution has not been achieved.

STAGE 1: LOCAL RESOLUTION

For a complaint to be investigated under the complaints procedure, it must originate within a year of either the event or the complainant becoming aware of a cause for complaint (date of knowledge). This time limit can be extended at the discretion of the complaints manager if there are mitigating circumstances and it is still possible to investigate the complaint fully and fairly. Complaints can be made to the individual or organisation providing the service or to the commissioning body but not both and can be made verbally, by email or by letter. They can be instigated by either the patient or a third party acting on their behalf, including relatives, solicitors or others such as their local MP. The representative must have the written consent of the patient, unless the patient is:

- Deceased, in which case the complainant must be their personal representative, i.e. an executor of the will or someone with a Lasting Power of Attorney (LPA) for healthcare matters (see Chapter 16).
- Someone who lacks the capacity to consent and the complaint is in their best interests (see Chapter 5).
- A non-Gillick competent child and the complaint is in their best interests (see Chapter 5).

Local authorities have a statutory duty to provide independent advocacy services to assist people with making complaints against the NHS regarding their care or treatment and they must be given this information at the earliest possible stage.

All responsible bodies must have a complaints manager accessible to the public and a 'responsible person', who ensures compliance with the complaint processes and must sign all responses to complaints. They should publicise their complaints procedures to both staff and patients and provide explanatory leaflets. Note that hospitals may have more than one complaints manager and in general practices, the role is often delegated to the practice manager, which may lead to conflict, especially where the manager is an employee of the person being complained about. Where the complaint relates to more than one responsible body, they have a statutory 'duty to cooperate' and must work together to provide a single agreed response.

The emphasis should be on the rapid and preferably informal resolution of complaints. Members of staff are encouraged to deal with complaints as they arise, but they should refer any that they believe warrant further investigation or where they do not feel that they can provide adequate reassurance to the complainant. These complaints should be investigated by the complaints manager on behalf of either the chief executive or the senior principal of the practice, in accordance with the following time scales:

- **Acknowledgement**: Complaints must be acknowledged in writing by an identified claims handler within 3 days and include a summary of the complaint with offers to discuss both the handling of the complaint and the time frame for response. It must also provide the complainant with information about the local NHS Complaint Advocacy Services. Note that if it is not possible to meet the time frame identified, the complainant must be kept fully informed of the delay and the underlying reasons. Where possible, oral complaints should be resolved within 24 hours and if the patient is satisfied with the response, formal written acknowledgement is not necessary. The complaint and response should be documented and stored in a complaint file held separately from the clinical notes. If oral complaints cannot be resolved within 24 hours, they must be handled in the same way as written ones.
- **Investigation**: Following the investigation, the provider of care or service must issue a response to NHS England. For clinical complaints, this response will be evaluated by an appropriate peer clinical reviewer, independently appointed by NHS England, e.g. the response to a complaint about a GP will be subject to review by an independent GP. A similar process is also used for contractual issues and complaints about due process.
- **Response**: This must be sent either by or on behalf of the senior partner in a primary care practice or the Chief Executive of the Trust. It must contain an explanation of how the complaint was considered, including details of any reference materials used to help reach the decision such as reports and guidelines, details of personnel involved in the investigation and the reasons for the final conclusion. It should provide a meaningful apology where appropriate and information about steps taken to rectify any areas found lacking. It

must be sent within 40 days and if it is likely to take more than 6 months, the complainant must be updated with the reasons for the delay and likely date of resolution. The complainant should also be signposted to the second stage involving the PHSO, should they be dissatisfied with the response.

STAGE 2: PARLIAMENTARY HEALTH SERVICE OMBUDSMAN

If a complainant is not satisfied with the response following local resolution, he can refer his complaint to the PHSO for the second stage of the procedure. The PHSO can also consider grievances about the complaints process. The post of PHSO is a Crown appointment and the Office is entirely independent of both the Government and the NHS, although the PHSO is accountable to Parliament. It combines the two statutory roles of the Parliamentary Commissioner for Administration (the Parliamentary Ombudsman) and the Health Service Commissioner for England (Health Service Ombudsman). The powers and jurisdiction of the Office are governed by the *Parliamentary Commissioner Act 1967* and the *Health Service Commissioners Act 1993*, as amended in 1996 to allow the Ombudsman to investigate complaints related to clinical judgement.

The complainant must be the aggrieved party, his personal representative or a family member. It cannot be a public authority. The complaint must be in writing and the incident should have occurred within the past year unless there are mitigating factors, but the PHSO can decide to investigate complaints older than 12 months if he deems it appropriate. The PHSO has the same rights of access to persons and documents as the High Court, but the investigations must be done in private.

The PHSO will consider all cases on their merits but will only order a further investigation if there is evidence of a service failure, not just because the complainant is unhappy with the outcome. He is required to investigate complaints of hardship or injustice as a consequence of:

1. Failure in a service provided by a health service body
2. Failure of such a body to provide a service
3. Maladministration connected with any other action taken or on behalf of such a body
4. Clinical complaints following events arising on or after 1 April 1996.

Examples of such complaints include waiting lists, poor communication, cancellation of operations, confidentiality issues and handling of complaints.

The PHSO cannot investigate complaints:

1. Those have not been through the NHS complaints procedure
2. Where litigation is in process
3. Where the patient has a remedy in a court or before a tribunal, unless the PHSO believes that it would be unreasonable to expect the complainant to take that option
4. About private healthcare, unless it was funded by the NHS
5. Relating to NHS contracts—either with staff or with other bodies, e.g. cleaning.

If the PHSO decides not to investigate a complaint, he must write to the complainant and explain why.

Clinical complaints are reviewed by clinical advisers to the PHSO. If they consider that the management is not open to criticism, the PHSO will advise the complainant that there will be no intervention, giving the reasons for doing so. If there are grounds for questioning the clinical judgement, then the case will be investigated using external professional assessors from the relevant specialty. The investigation may be based solely on the notes but can involve interviews with the relevant staff. The investigators then produce a report of their findings, which takes the form of a peer review, using the 'Bolam' standard (see Chapter 9). The PHSO then reports in confidence to the complainant, the organisation and anyone against whom the complaint was made.

If the PHSO finds that there has been a deficiency in the actions of either an individual practitioner or an NHS body, he will ask them to agree to an apology being conveyed to the complainant in the report. If he considers that remedial action is required, he will recommend it. He actually has no power to force either an apology or a remedial action but in practice, most accept the recommendations. There is no appeal procedure if either party is dissatisfied with the report—the only redress available is a judicial review.

The PHSO aims to complete all investigations within 3 to 6 months and although complex investigations may take longer, 95% should be completed within a year. About 50% of cases are at least partially upheld.

NHS COMPLAINTS PROCEDURE IN SCOTLAND

The NHS complaints procedure in Scotland is a two-stage process similar to that in England but it is governed by the *Patient Rights (Scotland) Act 2011*, and if the local resolution procedure is not successful, patients can complain directly to the Scottish Public Services Ombudsman (SPSO). The complaints manager is called the 'feedback and complaints officer' and a complaint must be made within 6 months of the occurrence or date of knowledge, not a year. Although this can be flexible, the SPSO can only investigate complaints more than 1 year old in exceptional circumstances. Initial acknowledgement should be within 3 working days with a full response within 20 days.

NHS COMPLAINTS PROCEDURE IN WALES

In Wales, the NHS complaints procedure is also a two-stage process, but it is covered by the *NHS (Concerns, Complaints & Redress Arrangements) (Wales) Regulations 2011*, and if the local resolution procedure fails, patients can complain directly to the Public Services Ombudsman for Wales. The regulations refer to 'concerns', which include complaints, adverse incidents and dissatisfaction, and there is also a redress component where if there is 'qualifying liability', patients can be offered up to £25,000 in financial redress. Note that the redress requirement only applies to Welsh NHS hospitals and local health boards, not primary or private care providers of NHS services. Concerns can be raised in the same way as complaints in the English system, but the regulations also allow staff to notify concerns about patient care. The time limit is again 1 year from the incident or date of knowledge but no more than 3 years. Hospitals and practices must appoint a 'responsible officer' to oversee the process and a 'senior investigations manager' to deal with the concerns. Initial acknowledgement should be within 2 working days with a full response within 30 days.

NHS COMPLAINTS PROCEDURE IN NORTHERN IRELAND

The NHS complaints procedure in Northern Ireland is also a two-stage process, which must comply with the *Complaints in Health & Social Care: Standards & Guidelines for Resolution & Learning 2009* and in the second stage, patients can apply to the Northern Ireland Public Services Ombudsman. Complaints must be brought within 6 months of the incident or date of knowledge and they are investigated by a complaints manager.

WHY PATIENTS COMPLAIN

In 2005/2006, there were 95,047 written complaints about NHS services, but this had more than doubled to 208,626 by 2017/2018.[1] The number continues to rise but it seems to relate to changes in patient expectations and acceptance, as there is no evidence to suggest that the number of mistakes made by healthcare professionals (HCPs) has risen. Factors that have been shown to influence the number of complaints include the involvement of the Patients Advice and Liaison Service (PALS) and the success rate of local organisations in resolving issues when they first arise.[2] In 2018/2019, approximately 58.4% of complaints were made against hospitals and community health services and about 52% of those against GP and dental primary care services were upheld or partially upheld.[3] Note that the Patient's Charter actively encourages patients to provide feedback and complain if they are dissatisfied, theoretically to improve the service, and advises them of their right to an investigation and a written reply.

The following are the commonest sources of complaint:
1. 'All aspects' of clinical treatment but particularly communication
2. Staff attitudes, especially if there was a perceived lack of respect
3. Delays and cancellation of outpatient appointments
4. Missed, delayed or incorrect diagnosis.

The reasons that patients give for bringing the complaint include:
- Acknowledgement that there has been a problem
- Wanting answers or an apology
- Needing assurance that what has happened to themselves or to a relative will not happen to others
- Wanting to know what remedial actions, if any, will be taken to prevent such an event from happening again
- Wanting financial compensation
- Wanting the member(s) of staff involved to be punished.

RESPONDING TO A COMPLAINT
- If you receive a formal complaint, you must discuss it with your complaints manager before any action. You have the right to be involved in the response and if you do not feel that your comments are being fairly represented, you should speak to your indemnity provider.
- If you are asked to respond to a complaint, you must investigate the complaint thoroughly, ensuring that you have a clear understanding of the issues raised, the circumstances and the outcome that the complainant wants. This should include interviews

with all the staff involved and taking statements where necessary. You should also perform a comprehensive review of the notes and assess the situation at the time of the complaint, e.g. if the complaint involves an attendance at the Emergency Department, then you should also consider the staffing levels, waiting times, number of attendances and the case mix. Have a clear plan for your investigation with an estimate of the likely timescales and consider who should review the complaint. Ensure that at all times, you respect the confidentiality of all patient-related information (see Chapter 6), particularly if the complaint has been brought by a third party.
- Be prompt in your reply—bear in mind the time limits and keep the complainant updated about any delays and the reasons for them.
- Include an expression of regret that the complainant was unhappy with the service provided.
- Be open and honest and apologise where it is appropriate but do not try to defend situations beyond your control, e.g. inadequate staffing levels. Remember that saying sorry is NOT an admission of liability—Section 2 of the *Compensation Act 2006* states 'an apology, an offer of treatment or other redress, shall not of itself amount to an admission of negligence or breach of statutory duty'.
- Describe in detail the circumstances that contributed to the complaint, e.g. waiting times.
- If other parties are also involved, ensure that you have received a report from them and that they are aware that you are replying to the complaint on their behalf.
- Provide a factual reply that specifically addresses **all** the points made in the complaint and each point should preferably be enumerated.
- **Never** be defensive or appear hostile towards the complainant.
- If practice has changed as a result of the complaint in an effort to prevent a recurrence, tell the complainant as this may be all they wanted.
- Inform the complainant of their right to go to the PHSO within 12 months if they are dissatisfied with the response and of the support services available, such as PALS.
- Be aware of the possibility that the complaint is simply an exercise in gathering information for future litigation.
- Complaints are often an opportunity to remind the management that there are deficiencies in the service provided that need to be addressed such as inadequate facilities or supervision of junior staff.

DUTY OF CANDOUR

Regulation 20 of the *Health & Social Care Act 2008 (Regulated Activities) Regulations 2014* made the professional duty of candour a legal requirement of every HCP working for health and adult social care providers registered with the Care Quality Commission (CQC) (see Chapter 7).

The duty of candour means that all HCPs must be open and honest with their patients, colleagues, employers and relevant organisations. They must participate in reviews and investigations when requested and they must raise concerns with their regulators, where appropriate. They must support and encourage each other to behave in the same manner and not stop someone else from raising concerns.

With special regard for patient care, if something goes wrong with their treatment or care and causes or has the potential to cause, harm or distress, the HCP must:

- tell the patient when an error has occurred or, where appropriate, their advocate, carer or family
- apologise to the patient or, where appropriate, their advocate, carer or family
- if possible, offer a suitable remedy or support to resolve matters
- provide a full explanation of the potential short- and long-term effects of what has happened to the patient or, where appropriate, their advocate, carer or family.

SUMMARY

This chapter outlines the two-stage complaints process from local resolution to referral to the Parliamentary Health Service Ombudsman and highlights the differences in the process within the different countries of the UK. It lists the reasons why patients complain and suggests why the number of complaints has increased over the years. It advises the reader about how best to respond to and investigate a complaint. It also defines the duty of candour and explains why it is now a statutory duty as well as an ethical one.

NOTES

1. NHS Digital, *Data on written complaints in the NHS, 2005-06*, 15 November 2006; NHS Digital, *Data on written complaints in the NHS, 2018-19*, 5 September 2019.
2. NHS Digital, *Data on written complaints in the NHS, 2018-19* (September 2019), p. 7.
3. NHS Digital, *Data on written complaints in the NHS, 2018-19*, Data Tables, T1b, 9.

FURTHER READING

NHS England Complaints Policy 2013, as updated 2021.

USEFUL WEBSITES

NHS Complaints: www.nhs.uk/using-the-nhs/about-the-nhs/how-to-complain-to-the-nhs

Parliamentary Health Service Commissioner: www.ombudsman.org.uk

Department of Health: www.open.gov.uk/doh

NHS Digital: www.digital.nhs.uk

CHAPTER 9

Clinical Negligence

DEFINITION OF CLINICAL NEGLIGENCE

In the United Kingdom, unless the negligence has been so gross as to amount to a criminal act, most cases of alleged clinical negligence are regarded as *torts* ('delicts' in Scotland) or civil wrongs and are dealt with through civil proceedings.

For an allegation of negligence by a healthcare professional (HCP) to succeed, the claimant ('pursuer' in Scotland) must prove all four of the following:
1. The defendant had a **duty of care** to the claimant
2. There was a **breach** of that duty of care
3. The claimant suffered **actionable harm or damage**
4. The damage was caused by the breach (**causation**).

DUTY OF CARE

All HCPs have a duty to become and remain competent at their job and they should be diligent in providing those skills to those who need them. The various professional bodies, such as the General Medical Council (GMC), Nursing and Midwifery Council (NMC) or Health and Care Professions Council (HCPC) (see Chapter 10) set the minimum standards necessary, but the level of skill and proficiency will vary with experience, continuing education and seniority. If a senior HCP delegates a task to a more junior one, he must be confident that his colleague has sufficient experience and skill to do it, as the senior still carries part,

if not all, responsibility for any resultant errors. This is known as **vicarious liability** and also applies to Trusts, who are held to be legally responsible for the actions of the staff that they employ (see Chapter 7). This overarching responsibility does **not** apply to allegations arising from 'Good Samaritan' acts or other activities such as the provision of statements or private medical reports, referrals to professional bodies, e.g. the GMC or voluntary work, so all HCPs should also have private indemnity insurance. General Practitioners are vicariously responsible for the staff who they employ, e.g. receptionists or nurses, but **not** for locums or deputising doctors. They are also responsible for any claims made against them so **must** have private indemnity insurance (see Chapter 7).

In some cases, it is obvious that the HCP owes a duty of care, e.g. a patient with a 'named nurse', those who are on the practice list or have paid a fee for a service. However, a duty of care can be legally established in other situations, such as a doctor stopping at a roadside to help following a car crash. In some countries, e.g. France, doctors must stop at the site of a car accident by law and can be prosecuted if it can be proved that they drove past, but in the United Kingdom, 'Good Samaritan' acts remain an ethical duty only.

If an HCP examines a patient for any purpose other than to provide advice or treatment, there is no established duty of care, e.g. insurance, drink-drive or pre-employment examinations. If the patient is harmed during the examination, then he is entitled to sue the HCP, but he cannot accuse him of negligence if he is refused insurance on the basis of the medical report. In such cases, the duty of the HCP is to the insurance company, not to the patient.

BREACH OF DUTY OF CARE

An HCP breaches his duty of care if he fails to reach the level of proficiency of his peers. This is known as the **Bolam Test** and it applies equally to the duty to treat, diagnose, gain informed consent and give advice. It follows the case of *Bolam v Friern Hospital Management Committee 1957*,[1] where the claimant was given electro-convulsive therapy without sedation or manual restraint and suffered bilateral hip fractures.

He sued the hospital for negligence, but the claim was dismissed on the basis that his management was the standard practice at that time. The judge, Justice McNair, said that a doctor was not negligent if he acted in accordance with a responsible and competent body of relevant professional opinion even if other doctors adopted a different practice. It is important to remember that courts retain the right to decide whether an established medical practice is acceptable, so it may not be sufficient to provide expert opinion to support a particular treatment. It should also be noted that in Scotland, the test case was that of *Hunter v Hanley*[2] and the ruling stated that a doctor had to act in accordance with a 'responsible doctor', so the standard is potentially lower.

Ignorance is no defence in negligence and the case of *Wilsher v Essex Area Health Authority*[3] ruled that the duty of care of a junior HCP includes an obligation to seek senior advice. Although a junior cannot be expected to have the same skills as a senior, the duty of care relates to the act and patients are entitled to optimum care, independent of the provider. If a junior does not have the skill or experience to proficiently perform a procedure, then he **must** defer to his senior.

2015 brought the first case of negligence based on 'flawed consent' following the case of *Mongomery*,[4] where the attending doctor was held to be negligent because she had not disclosed all 'material risks' or 'those to which a 'prudent patient' would have attached significance' (see Chapter 5). This ruling has been criticised[5] in that it may be difficult to know what risks would be especially significant to a particular patient, but it does highlight the guidance from all the professional bodies that good communication should underpin every patient–HCP relationship.

Note that genuine errors of clinical judgement are not the same as negligence. All HCPs make mistakes but if they can show that they exercised reasonable skill and care in coming to their decision, then they cannot be held to have been negligent, even if that decision was wrong, e.g. an incorrect diagnosis or treatment. The breach can be either something:

1. done (commission), e.g. forceps left in the chest after heart surgery
2. not done (omission), e.g. failure to attend to a sick patient or to obtain fully informed consent.

ACTIONABLE HARM OR DAMAGE

This is the disability, loss or injury suffered by the claimant and it is distinct from 'damages', which is the financial compensation awarded to a successful claimant. However negligent the defendant has been, the claimant must have suffered **quantifiable harm** as a result for the action to be successful, e.g. if a doctor delays in diagnosing a particular condition, then he is only negligent if the delay adversely affects the final outcome. Quantifiable harm (quantum) includes loss of earnings, reduced quality or quantity of life, disfigurement, disability and mental anguish.

There may also be an element of **contributory negligence**, where the actions of the claimant are judged to have made the situation worse, e.g. removing a dressing or failing to attend follow-up appointments. This does not affect the judgement but can reduce the amount of damages awarded. If the claimant was off work as a result of the injury and received Social Security benefits such as Statutory Sick Pay, under the *Social Security Administration Act 1992*, an amount equal to the benefits is subtracted from the compensation payment. The corresponding provision in Northern Ireland is the *Social Security Administration (Northern Ireland) Act 1992*. These Acts apply to injuries or diseases that occurred after 1 January 1989 and the deduction is paid directly to the Department of Social Security by the compensator. If the injury occurred before 1 January 1989, then the compensator keeps the deduction. There are some exemptions such as payments of £2500 or less, those made under the *Vaccine Damage Payments Act 1979* or those from the Criminal Injuries Compensation Board.

CAUSATION

Causation is the link between the actionable harm and the breach of duty of care, i.e. on a balance of probabilities, it is more likely that the harm suffered by the claimant resulted from the actions of the defendant. This is also known as the 'but for' test—the harm would not have happened 'but for' the actions of the HCP. An important case is that of *Bolitho*,[6] where the child died from a hypoxic brain injury that may have been avoided had he been intubated. The doctor was held to have breached her duty of care by not attending the child, but she was not found to be negligent in that she said that had she seen the patient, she would not have intubated him, as that was not the standard practice at that time, so the actionable harm would not have been avoided. As such, there was no link between the breach and the harm, so causation could not be established and the case was dismissed. Because negligence cases are decided on probability, causation is seen in law as binary and if the chance of something happening is over 50%, then it is assumed that it would have happened. In the case of *Gregg v Scott*,[7] the delay in the diagnosis of cancer by Dr Scott decreased Mr Gregg's chances of surviving from 42% to 25% but the claim was dismissed because his original chance of survival was under 50%. This failure to recognise medical uncertainty may mean that future cases will be decided on 'loss of a chance' and possibility rather than probability.

THE LEGAL PROCESS

The burden of proof is on the claimant, i.e. he must prove that the defendant has been negligent and the standard of proof is the civil standard, i.e. the *balance of probabilities* (see Chapter 2). The only exceptions are cases where the facts are so obvious that the onus is on the HCP to prove that he was not negligent, e.g. amputation of the wrong foot. This is the doctrine of *res ipsa loquitur* ('the facts speak for themselves') and these almost invariably settle out of court.

Due to the *Limitation Act 1980*, actions for negligence must be brought within 3 years of **the date of knowledge**, which is either the date on which the alleged negligence occurred or when the patient became aware of the effects, which may be years later. There are exceptions to this rule—if the claimant was mentally ill at the time of the injury, it starts at the date of recovery or if he was a child, there is no time limit. The court can also allow cases out of time to proceed if it would not prejudice either party to do so—one case was settled for £1.25m 33 years after the original damage to his brain that occurred during birth. This means that it is often very difficult to defend negligence cases and emphasises the importance of making good contemporaneous notes.

Following the introduction of the Civil Procedure Rules (CPR) in 1997, both parties must follow the Pre-action Protocol developed by the Clinical Disputes Forum. This has a *commitments* section, which sets out the principles that both the healthcare provider and the patient should follow. For the healthcare provider, these are essentially the same as those for clinical risk management (see Chapter 7), while the patient has an obligation to bring any concerns to the healthcare provider as early as possible. He must also consider all the options available, including negotiation and the complaints procedures (see Chapter 8) before starting litigation. The *steps* section sets out a recommended sequence of actions to be followed if litigation is in prospect and the process is given in Fig. 9.1.

COST OF CLINICAL NEGLIGENCE

Despite improvements in the safety and quality of clinical care, the number of negligence claims is increasing. In 2019–2020, NHS Resolution (see Chapter 7) reported 11,682 new clinical claims and the annual cost of harm due to clinical activity was £8.3 billion. The cost of settling claims was £2.9 billion, although the majority were settled out of court with only 0.6% going to trial. The majority were low value but while obstetric cases only accounted for 10% of the number of claims, they were responsible for about 50% of the cost.[8]

There is also the emotional cost to both the clinician and the patient, as clinical negligence cases can be long and stressful. There may be professional implications too, so all HCPs are advised to have personal indemnity insurance.

NO FAULT COMPENSATION

In some countries such as Sweden and New Zealand, claimants need to only show that the injury resulted from 'medical or surgical misadventure' and compensation is based on need. The claimant does not have to prove negligence by the HCP involved, but if the injury followed a complication, it may be difficult to show that it was so rare as to constitute a misadventure, i.e. not avoidable through the exercise of reasonable care. It is also often hard to distinguish between the consequence of treatment and the natural progress of the disease.

THE ROLE OF THE MEDICAL EXPERT WITNESS

The outcome of a medical negligence case often depends upon the quality of the evidence from the medical expert witness(es), so it is a crucial role. Medical expert witnesses should have at least 10 to 15 years' experience in their field, with a good reputation and respected by their peers. Their role is to consider the facts of the case, answer any questions, clarify any clinical terms or descriptions for the court and provide an accurate, independent and impartial opinion based on their qualifications and experience. Their evidence may be oral and/or written and based on notes, oral evidence or on their own examination of the patient.

CRIMINAL NEGLIGENCE

Although more common than previously, criminal convictions for negligence are still very rare and

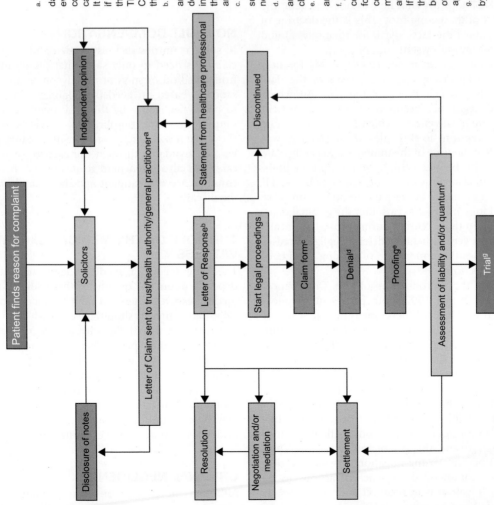

a. The Letter of Claim informs the recipient of the dates of the alleged negligent treatment and the events giving rise to the claim. It also details the injuries, condition and future prognosis, with an outline of the causal link between the injuries and the allegations. It may also include a request for the medical notes if they have not already been provided, the likely value of the claim and an offer to settle. The defendant must acknowledge the Letter of Claim within 14 days and provide copies of the requested records within 40 days.

b. The Letter of Response must be provided within 4 months and should comment on the events if they are disputed, with details of any other documentation upon which the defendant intends to rely. If breach of duty and causation are accepted, then suggestions may be made regarding resolution and/or settlement.

c. Civil courts issue claim forms instead of writs or originating summons. They contain 'particulars of claim' and 'particulars of negligence'.

d. The defendant must specify the reasons for any denial and state his own version of events if it differs from that of the claimant.

e. 'Proofing' means that the defendant's solicitors prepare answers to the particulars.

f. Assessment of quantum means that the level of financial compensation is estimated based on previous settlements for similar injuries and standard textbooks. If it is likely to cost more to defend the case than to settle, the defendant may consider this to be the better option, although there is an implication of guilt that will then not be contested. If the Trust is defending the action and decides to settle, the HCP(s) involved will probably not be consulted and may be left feeling that justice has not been served. Assessment of liability means that all the evidence is considered, and if it appears that the defendant is liable, then the case is settled.

g. Only a small minority of cases go to court and are decided by the judge on the basis of expert opinion.

FIG. 9.1 Steps in the legal process following a complaint.

effectively limited to prosecutions for manslaughter. In *R v Bateman*,[9] the judge stressed that for criminal liability to be established, the negligence must go beyond compensation to such disregard for life and safety as to amount to a crime against the State. Gross negligence manslaughter was first defined in the case of *R v Adomako*,[10] where an anaesthetist failed to recognise that the endotracheal tube had become disconnected and the patient was in distress. There was conflicting evidence to suggest that he was either present and grossly incompetent or not actually in the theatre, having left the patient without adequate monitoring. The patient died and Dr Adomako was convicted of manslaughter, although his sentence was suspended. In a more recent case, a trainee paediatrician, Dr Bawa-Garba, was convicted of gross negligence manslaughter following the death of a seriously ill 6-year-old boy in her care and was given a 2-year suspended sentence.[11] Note that in New Zealand, an HCP can be found criminally liable merely for failing to exercise 'reasonable knowledge, skill and care'.

SUMMARY

This chapter defines clinical negligence and outlines the components that must be present for a case of negligence to succeed—there must be a duty of care to the patient, a breach of that duty of care and actionable harm or damage as a direct result of that breach (causation). The differences between civil and criminal negligence are discussed and the legal process is demonstrated with a useful flowchart. The role of the medical expert witness is also considered and the importance of having private medical indemnity insurance is stressed throughout.

NOTES

1. *Bolam v Friern Management Committee* [1957] 2 All ER 118
2. *Hunter v Hanley* [1955] SC 200.
3. *Wilsher v Essex Area Health Authority* [1986] 3 All ER 801 (CA); [1988] 1 All ER 871 (HL).
4. *Montgomery v Lanarkshire Health Board* [2015] SC 11; [2015] 1 AC 1430.
5. Cyna, A.M., Simmons, S.W. Guidelines on informed consent in anaesthesia: unrealistic unethical, untenable. *Br J Anaesth.* 2017;119:1086–1089.
6. *Bolitho v City and Hackney Health Authority* [1997] UKHL 46; [1998] AC 232; [1997] 4 All ER 771; [1997] 3 WLR 1151.
7. *Gregg v Scott* [2005] UKHL 2.
8. See www.resolution.nhs.uk/2020/07/16/nhs-resolutions-annual-report-and-accounts-2019-20.
9. *R v Bateman* [1925] All ER Rep 45 at 48.
10. *R v Adomako* [1991] 2 Med LR 277.
11. *R v Bawa-Garba* [2016] EWCA Crim 184.

USEFUL WEBSITES

Citizens Advice Bureau: www.citizensadvice.org.uk/health/nhs-and-social-care-complaints

Action Against Medical Accidents: www.avma.org.uk

Disciplinary Bodies and Procedures

INTRODUCTION

Regulation of standards varies between the different healthcare professions from statutory disciplinary proceedings to guidelines, but the Councils discussed in this chapter do set standards to which the healthcare professional (HCP) must adhere and have disciplinary procedures for those who fail to do so. The original concept of 'self-regulation' by the various professional bodies led to increasing public concern, and although it has now changed to 'professional regulation', the structure and function of all three Councils are constantly under review.

THE GENERAL MEDICAL COUNCIL (GMC)

The GMC and the medical register were established by the *Medical Act 1858*. The GMC is an independent statutory body that is responsible for medical registration, regulation, education and discipline in the United Kingdom. It gains its current powers from the *Medical Act 1983* and there are 12 Council members, who oversee the work of the GMC and set the strategy and goals. Fifty percent are lay members and all are appointed by the Privy Council.

The functions of the GMC are as follows:

The Medical Register

The GMC maintains the medical register that allows all doctors to be identified for legal and official purposes and there are currently over 350,000 doctors registered in the United Kingdom. It gives the doctor's full name, date of birth, primary and any higher qualifications. It also states whether they hold a license to practise and if they are on either the Specialist or General Practitioner (GP) Register. The types of registration are as follows:

- **Provisional**—This only allows doctors to work in an approved UK Foundation Year 1 post—it cannot be used for anything else.
- **Full**—All doctors must be fully registered to work in an approved UK Foundation Year 2 post or in unsupervised medical practice.
- **Specialist**—In 1996, the GMC was required to establish a Specialist Register under the *European Specialist Medical Qualifications order 1995* and inclusion on the list is determined by the Specialist Training Authority. Inclusion depends on the successful completion of either 5 or 6 years training in a specialty, with yearly assessments and, for some specialties, fulfilment of an 'exit' examination. Most doctors working in the United Kingdom at a Consultant level in a medical or surgical specialty will hold a license to practice and full specialist registration, but this does not apply to locums.
- **GP**—Since 2006, all GPs working in the United Kingdom including locums must be on the GP register and on a GP Performers list unless they are trainees or GP Registrars.

Education

The GMC regulates and sets the standards for all providers of medical training and education. It also decides the outcomes that both medical students and trainee doctors should achieve by the end of their training. The role includes coordination of all the stages of medical education, curriculum changes and inspection of qualifying examinations from all examining bodies, including the Royal Colleges and medical schools. The GMC also supplies guidance and support hubs for areas such as reflective practice and revalidation.

Ethical Guidance

The GMC provides advice to doctors on medical ethics and professional standards through online resources and publications. It outlines the knowledge, skills, behaviours and professional values expected of all doctors working in the United Kingdom.

Revalidation

Recommendations from the fifth report into the case of Harold Shipman[1] to make professional self-regulation more transparent and accountable led the GMC to introduce the process of revalidation and now every registered doctor with a license to practice in the United Kingdom must revalidate every 5 years. Registered nurses must revalidate every 3 years (see NMC) and the professions regulated by the Health and Care Professions Council (HCPC) must all reregister every 2 years (see 'Health and Care Professions Council (HCPC)').

Doctors must show that they have a connection to a Responsible Officer (RO) or Suitable Person and belong to a Designated Body (DB), who appoints their RO and is usually their main place of employment. Doctors must undergo an annual appraisal by an approved appraiser and are required to collate a portfolio of evidence to support all areas of their scope of practice including continuing professional development (CPD), quality improvement activities and a record of complaints and compliments. The results of the appraisal are reported to the RO, who is responsible for:

- Evaluating the Fitness to Practice (FTP) of all doctors with a prescribed connection to the DB and making recommendations for revalidation to the GMC
- Ensuring that effective procedures are in place to support revalidation, including systems for appraisal and clinical governance (see Chapter 7)
- Overseeing doctors subject to supervised or restricted practices
- Providing measures for the effective support and remediation of doctors whose performance has fallen below the acceptable standard.

Disciplinary Procedures and Complaints Handling

Most complaints to the GMC are closed without any impact on the doctors' registration but it is a very stressful and protracted process that can have quite serious adverse effects on both the doctor's physical and mental health. The GMC considered 8468 FTP enquiries in 2020 and over 7000 were closed at the triage stage, as they either did not meet the threshold or related to matters that the GMC do not investigate. Six thousand three hundred and eighteen were raised by members of the public and 580 came from 'persons acting in a public capacity', which are primarily the police

and employers. The police are required to notify the GMC if a doctor is convicted of **any** criminal offence and offences involving personal conduct, e.g. misuse of alcohol or drugs, dishonesty, indecency, fraud or violence. Other sources include the media, fellow doctors and self-referral. The GMC will only investigate concerns relating to events that occurred less than 5 years earlier unless there is likely to be public interest in the case.

There are several stages to the complaints handling process:

- **Triage**
  This is done to establish whether the doctor's FTP is in question. Those not related to FTP, e.g. a contested decision on an insurance report, are closed immediately. Complaints that raise concerns but do not warrant a full investigation will be referred to the employer or RO (see 'Revalidation') unless there is a pattern of behaviour.
- **Provisional enquiries**
  Since 2014, the GMC has conducted provisional enquiries following triage and over 70% of cases close before a full investigation.
- **Investigation**
  If the GMC decides to investigate a concern, they will write to the practitioner with details of the allegation(s) and invite a written response within 28 days to address the concern(s) and provide any additional evidence. They will also inform his employer or sponsoring body. The GMC expects the doctor to show insight into the gravity of the concerns raised and demonstrate that they have taken remedial action to address them. This is called 'remediation' and can have a positive impact on the eventual outcome of the case. Doctors must engage with the GMC as part of their obligations under 'Good Medical Practice',[2] but they are advised to speak to their medical indemnity provider before replying, as the GMC will only open an investigation if they believe that they may need to restrict the practice of the doctor if the concern is proven. Grounds for a full investigation include:
  - Misconduct
  - A criminal caution or conviction
  - Poor performance
  - Physical or mental ill-health that may or does impact performance e.g. drug or alcohol dependence
  - Inadequate command of English
  - A decision by anther regulatory body, either in the United Kingdom or abroad

The GMC investigators will gather evidence, including statements, medical notes and expert reports and they should complete their investigation within a year. If they consider that the concern warrants immediate restriction or suspension or if it involves a serious criminal conviction, the doctor will be referred straight to the Medical Practitioners Tribunal Service (MPTS—see later) for an Interim Orders Tribunal. Depending on the nature of the concern, they may also require one or more of the following assessments:

- **Performance assessment:** The standard of the doctor's professional knowledge, skills and attitude towards patients and colleagues is assessed by a team of independent performance assessors. This includes peer reviews, visits to the doctor's work and both knowledge-based and practical tests. The doctor is given the opportunity to comment on both the assessment and the outcome.
- **Health assessment:** Where there are concerns about the doctor's health, the GMC can invite him to be examined by two independent medical examiners. They will assess both his physical and mental health and produce a report, stating the likely impact, if any, on his FTP and any recommendations, e.g. supervised or limited practice.
- **English language assessment:** The doctor must pass either the *International English Language Testing System* (*IELTS*) test or the *Occupational English Test* (*OET*).
- **Decision by case examiners**

There are usually two senior case examiners, one medical and one lay and they can make the following decisions:
  - Take no further action.
  - Issue a *warning*—this is used if the doctors' performance has been shown to be below the acceptable standard and should not be repeated but does not warrant any restrictions. The warning and a summary of the case will only remain on the Medical Register for 2 years, but they are kept on record after that time and can be disclosed to future employers on request. If the doctor refuses to accept the warning, he will be referred to the Investigation Committee who can either place the warning on the Register, conclude the case with no further action or refer the doctor to the MPTS.

- Agree an *undertaking* with the doctor—these include refraining from doing certain things, retraining or being supervised.
- Refer the doctor to the MPTS for a full tribunal hearing.

THE MEDICAL PRACTITIONERS TRIBUNAL SERVICE

Formed in 2012, the MPTS is a statutory committee of the GMC, but it is operationally separate and has different accountability. It adjudicates on complaints to make independent decisions about a doctor's FTP through both **Interim Orders Tribunals (IOTs)** and **FTP Tribunals**. It is based in Manchester and there are 16 hearing rooms.

Doctors are referred to the MPTS for the following reasons:
- If proven, the allegations suggest such a serious failure to meet GMC standards that their FTP must be impaired. Examples include:
  - violence
  - sexual assault or indecency
  - practising without a license
  - inappropriate sexual or emotional relationships
  - gross negligence
  - dishonesty
  - unlawful discrimination.
- A conviction (other than minor, e.g. parking offences), caution or a determination from another regulatory body
- Refusal to agree to undertakings.

If the GMC investigation raises concerns of serious risks to patients or others, the case can be referred to the **IOT** at any stage. The IOT can decide that the doctor should be suspended or placed under conditions such as supervised practice to protect patients while the investigation continues. Their decision must be reviewed every 6 months and usually remains in place for up to 18 months, but it can be extended by a High Court order.

FTP tribunals have three members of which at least one must be medical and one lay and most hearings will have a legally qualified Chair to advise on points of law. Hearings are held in public and witnesses may be compelled to appear. Oral evidence is given on oath and the practitioner is entitled to legal representation. The doctor can dispute and rebut evidence and impairment must be *proved by evidence* unless the doctor admits it. The tribunal must also consider testimonials and the past history of the doctor.

There are three stages:

1. All the evidence is heard and the panel must decide to the criminal standard of *beyond reasonable doubt* (see Chapter 2) whether the facts have been proved. If they have,
2. The panel must decide if the doctor's FTP is impaired *at the time of the hearing*, so they must consider any remediation and if the doctor has taken successful steps to reform. A GMC study found that doctors who apologised and showed insight were much less likely to be erased. If his FTP is impaired, then
3. The panel must decide on the appropriate sanction, if any, and they can:
   - Take no action
   - Issue a warning, even if his FTP was not proved to be impaired
   - Agree to undertakings offered by the doctor at the hearing
   - Impose conditions on registration
   - Suspend the doctor for a set period of time
   - Erase him from the register.

In 2019, there were 257 FTP tribunals—120 doctors were suspended and 55 were erased. Doctors have a right of appeal within 28 days to the High Court in England and Wales, the Court of Session in Scotland or the High Court of Justice in Northern Ireland. The practitioner continues on the Register until appeal if it is granted unless there has been an order made for immediate suspension. Following changes to the *Medical Act 1983* in 2015, the GMC has also been able to appeal decisions made by the MPTS to the High Court if they consider them to be too lenient and there are concerns for patient safety.

THE NURSING AND MIDWIFERY COUNCIL (NMC)

The NMC replaced the UKCC in 2002 and it is both a statutory body established through the *Nursing and Midwifery Order 2001* and a charity, registered under the *Charities Commission*. It regulates all nurses and midwives in the United Kingdom and all nursing associates (NA) in England. It is run by the NMC Council, who are responsible for overseeing the NMC staff and establishing the strategic direction of the NMC. The Council has 12 lay and registrant members, with four representing each of the UK countries and they are appointed by the Privy Council. There is also a Midwifery Panel, which meets four times a year and reports to the Council. The functions of the NMC are as follows.

Maintenance of the Register

The NMC maintains the register of nurses, midwives and NA in a similar fashion to the GMC and all must be on the register to practice in the United Kingdom. The register provides details of nurses, midwives and NA who are:

- Currently fully registered with no restrictions or cautions
- Registered but with a caution order or restrictions to practice
- Have been suspended or erased since 2008 and are not currently allowed to practice.

All new nurses, midwives and NA in the United Kingdom must register following the successful completion of their course and pay the registration fee, which is currently £120. If they delay by more than 6 months, they must also provide a professional reference. Those who have trained outside the United Kingdom must complete an eligibility and qualification application and take a professional competence test before registering. Nursing staff can also apply for readmission following, e.g. a career break or restoration following erasure. The practitioner has a right to apply for restoration at any time, but it is unlikely to be considered for less than 1 year or until the specified period has elapsed and if removal followed conviction for a serious criminal offence, then restoration is very unlikely. In order to be restored, the practitioner must show that he:

1. understands and accepts the reason for his removal
2. has taken appropriate action to address the problem
3. has been working in a related field for a significant time period with exemplary conduct and impeccable references.

There is an appeals process whereby unsuccessful registration appeals are heard by an Appeals panel at a public hearing.

Setting Standards

The NMC produces the *Code*,[3] which sets out the professional standards of practice and behaviour to which nurses, midwives and NA must adhere to remain registered with the NMC. It was last updated in 2015 and it is against this that complaints of misconduct are judged. There are four main sections:

- Prioritise people
- Practice effectively
- Preserve safety
- Promote professionalism and trust.

Education

Like the GMC, the NMC regulates and sets the standards for all providers of nursing and midwifery training and education.

Revalidation

Nurses, midwives and NA must revalidate every 3 years and meet the following revalidation requirements to show that they are adhering to the principles of the *Code*:

- 450 practice hours
- 35 hours of CPD
- 5 pieces of practice-related feedback
- 5 written reflective accounts
- A reflective discussion
- A health and character declaration
- Evidence of current professional indemnity
- Confirmation—this is the process by which the practitioner demonstrates to an 'appropriate person' (usually their manager) that they have met the revalidation requirements and it is completed in the final year of each 3-year cycle.

All the information is then submitted online directly to the NMC.

Management of Complaints and Disciplinary Proceedings

The NMC has a statutory obligation to investigate and deal with allegations of misconduct or unfitness to practice. Complaints can come from any source, but they must be in writing and sufficiently serious to justify either restrictions to practice or erasure from the register such as:

- abuse of position, e.g. inappropriate sexual relationships, bullying or discrimination
- violence, e.g. physical or verbal abuse of a patient
- dishonesty or fraud, e.g. stealing or falsifying records
- serious or repeated breaches in confidentiality or patient care.

As for the GMC, the police are required to notify the NMC if a registered nurse, midwife or NA is convicted of **any** criminal offence.

Complaints handling is similar to that of the GMC and involves several stages:

- **Screening**
  To pass on to the next stage, the concern must be in writing and it must be so serious as to warrant the need for regulatory action should it be proven. The evidence will also need to be examined to establish whether the nurse is safe to continue to practice or if he should be referred for an Interim Orders hearing. If they consider that the nurse is not fit to practice and the order is necessary to protect either the public and/or the practitioner, the panel can then impose either an interim suspension order or an interim conditions of practice order for up to 18 months. Interim orders must be reviewed every 6 months and can be extended by application to the High Court (Court of Session in Scotland).

- **Investigation**
  The NMC will write to the practitioner with details of the allegation(s) and invite a written response within 28 days to address the concern(s) and provide any additional evidence. They will also inform his employer or sponsoring body. Nursing staff must engage with the NMC as part of their obligations under the *Code*, but they are advised to speak to either the Royal College of Nursing (RCN) and/or their indemnity provider before replying. This process can take 25 weeks.

- **Case examiners' decisions**
  There are usually two case examiners, one lay and one nurse, midwife or NA according to the profession of the practitioner under investigation and they can make the following decisions:
  - Take no further action
  - Issue a *warning*—this remains on the register for 12 months
  - Agree an *undertaking* with the practitioner—these include supervised practice and extra or retraining
  - Referral to an FTP panel meeting or hearing.

- **FTP Committee meeting or hearing**
  FTP panels have three members of which at least one must be a nurse, midwife or NA of the same profession as the defendant and there will be an independent legal assessor to advise on points of law. At a meeting, the panel makes its decision solely on written evidence. There are no witnesses and the nurse under investigation cannot appear, although he can submit any further evidence that he wants the panel to consider. Hearings are held in public and witnesses may be compelled to appear. Oral evidence is given on oath and the practitioner is entitled to legal representation. At the conclusion, the panel can make the following decisions:
  - Take no action if the complaint has already been resolved
  - Issue a caution, which is placed on the register and can last from 1 to 5 years
  - Impose conditions on registration
  - Suspend the nurse for a set period of time
  - Erase him from the register.

HEALTH AND CARE PROFESSIONS COUNCIL (HCPC)

In 2003, the HCPC replaced the Council for Professions Supplementary to Medicine (CPSM) under the provisions of the *National Health Service Reform and Healthcare Professions Act 2002*. It provides a statutory framework for the registration, regulation, training and discipline of 15 health and care professions:

- Arts therapists
- Biomedical scientists
- Chiropodists/podiatrists
- Clinical scientists
- Dieticians
- Hearing aid dispensers
- Occupational therapists
- Operating department practitioners
- Orthoptists
- Paramedics
- Physiotherapists
- Practitioner psychologists
- Prosthetists and orthotists
- Radiographers
- Speech and language therapists.

In 2012, the HCPC also became responsible for the regulation of social workers, but in 2019, their regulation was transferred to Social Work England.

The functions of the HCPC are to:

- Set standards for education, training, conduct, performance and ethics for all the above professions
- Approve educational and training programmes and the qualifications necessary to become registered
- Maintain and publish the register
- Conduct all disciplinary procedures—anyone can raise a concern about a registrant's FTP including the public, his employer, colleagues or he can self-refer. Concerns include:
  - Misuse of title—each profession has one or more designated title, which is protected under the *Health Professions Order 2001* and it is a criminal offence to use it without being registered, to purport to be on the register when you are not or to falsely claim to have relevant qualifications
  - Impairment of FTP on the grounds of misconduct, incompetence, conviction/caution or mental or physical ill-health.

The HCPC cannot become involved in concerns raised about any of the following:

- nonregistrants
- organisations
- heath or social care arrangements
- issues that must be dealt with in court
- refunds or compensation.

HOSPITAL DISCIPLINARY PROCEDURES

In 2003, the Department of Health (DoH) brought in a new disciplinary framework for medical staff called *Maintaining High Professional Standards in the Modern NHS: a framework for the initial handling of concerns about doctors and dentists in the NHS*. It replaced the original procedure, which was mandated under Health Circular *HC(90)9 (Disciplinary procedures for Hospital and Community Medical and Dental Staff) 1990* and removed both the right of appeal to the Secretary of State and the Special Professional Panels (the 'three wise men'). Under the old rules, allegations of misconduct by HCPs were categorised into professional misconduct, personal misconduct and professional incompetence but this led to the 'suspension culture', where HCPs were excluded from work while they were being investigated due to a reluctance to use the standard disciplinary procedures. The current framework abolished the distinction between personal and professional misconduct, so HCPs were dealt with in the same way as other members of staff. It also introduced a new process for dealing with *capability issues*, relating to concerns about incompetence. It made the NHS employer solely responsible for disciplining staff in the hope that problems would be tackled earlier and improve standards, and it placed time limits on exclusion periods.

NHS employers have a duty to:

- Ensure that the disciplinary procedure is clearly stated in the written terms of employment and that it adheres to the *ACAS Code of Practice on Discipline and Grievance*
- Comply with the framework set out in the *Maintaining high professional standards in the modern NHS: a framework for the initial handling of concerns about doctors and dentists in the NHS*
- Carry out as full an investigation as possible in the given circumstances before taking any disciplinary action
- Inform all employees about the relevant appeal and grievance procedures.

In return, NHS employees must:

- Adhere to all codes of conduct and discipline within their terms of employment
- Co-operate with any disciplinary actions
- Follow the rules of any appeals or grievance procedures, even if they are no longer employed by the Trust.

Actions Once a Concern Has Been Raised

Allegations can come from any source including the HCP's fellow clinical staff, complaints from patients or relatives, a work incident, the revalidation process, quality improvement activities, audit, information from regulatory bodies, the coroner, the police or court judgements but all must be investigated.

The first step involves the line manager of the named HCP, who will first consider the seriousness of the allegation, with particular reference to patient safety, any possible criminality, probity, alcohol or drug misuse and anything that reaches the GMC or NMC thresholds for investigation, i.e. anything that if proven would affect the ability of the HCP to practice. Where appropriate, the line manager should involve the practitioner, HR and the Clinical or Medical Director. He should also seek advice from Practitioner Performance Advice (PPA) at NHS Resolution (see Chapter 7). The line manager should then conduct a fact-finding exercise to establish the dates and times of the incident, the staff involved and any witnesses. He will also gather other evidence such as rotas, medical notes and policies before examining all the evidence and any contributing or mitigating factors. If there is no evidence to support the allegation, there is no further action. If at any point of the disciplinary process the investigating officer finds that the HCP may present a danger to patient safety, then he must refer the HCP to either the GMC or NMC and consider exclusion or restricted practice (see later).

Informal Route

If the line manager decides that the misconduct has been minor and not part of a pattern of behaviour, he can take the informal route and talk directly to the HCP. He will advise of the correct standards that need to be met and can offer assistance such as retraining, coaching or supervised practice. This is known as an 'Improvement Conversation' and a written record is placed on the HCP's file. If he fails to improve, does not reach the standard within a set timescale or repeats the error, he will then be referred to the formal disciplinary route.

Formal Route

For more serious or repeated cases of misconduct, the Chief Executive will appoint a Case Manager to oversee the formal process. The Case Manager will then appoint a Case Investigator, who is usually an experienced HCP in the same specialty as the HCP under investigation. The HCP must be informed that he is being investigated and he can request a different Case Investigator if he believes that there would be a conflict of interest. He also has the right to see all the evidence and the list of witnesses if there is to be a hearing. At any stage, the HCP can be accompanied by a friend or a Union or indemnity insurance representative, but they cannot act in a legal capacity, unless it is at a hearing where the HCP is likely to be facing dismissal. The Case

Manager must also decide if there are grounds for the HCP to be excluded, but this should be a last resort. If the allegation also involves a police investigation, e.g. theft, then the disciplinary procedure can still proceed up to and including dismissal.

The Case Investigator should complete the report within 4 weeks and submit it to the Case Manager within a further 5 days but if it is likely to take longer, the practitioner should be kept informed at monthly intervals. The report should contain sufficient information to allow the Case Manager to decide if:
- There has been misconduct and the case should go before the professional conduct panel
- There are concerns about the health of the practitioner that should be referred to the occupational health department
- There are concerns about performance that need to be discussed with the PPA
- Exclusion or restrictions on practice should be considered
- There are serious concerns that warrant referral to the GMC or NMC
- The issues are so intractable that the case should be referred to the capability procedure
- No further action is required.

Disciplinary Hearing

If the Case Manager decides that there is a case to answer, there must be a disciplinary hearing before the professional conduct panel. The practitioner has the right to be informed in writing of the time, date and place, allegations, rights of representation and to bring his own witnesses. This must be at least 7 days in advance and he must also be provided with any documentary evidence and a list of witnesses. He can be accompanied by a representative, who can be a friend or someone from his Union or indemnity insurance provider. The representative can present the case on behalf of the HCP but cannot answer any questions. The Panel must include a member experienced in the same speciality as the HCP and the case is presented by the Chair, who starts by outlining the case and the nature of the allegations before calling any witnesses. The procedure is adversarial and interrogative and the defendant then states his case and calls any witnesses.

Once the hearing is concluded, the Panel decides on any disciplinary action and their decision must be confirmed in writing within 7 days, stating the rights of appeal. The following types of action are available:
1. Nothing proven and no action is taken.
2. **Formal first written warning**—the HCP has either failed to resolve the issue through the informal

approach or the misconduct was sufficiently serious to go straight to the formal procedure. This remains on record for a designated period, then lapses but it is usually for 6 months to 1 year.

3. **Formal final written warning**—this is for more than one serious offence in a year and/or continuing failure to meet standards and stays on the file for up to 18 months.

4. **Dismissal**—if the conduct remains unsatisfactory or constitutes gross misconduct, the HCP will be dismissed. This can either be with payment in lieu of notice or summary, which is immediate dismissal without notice, e.g. gross misconduct such as theft or assault or where the welfare of the patients has been put in jeopardy. This includes dereliction of duty and drug or alcohol abuse.

Appeals Against Disciplinary Sanctions

NHS employees have a right of appeal against any formal sanctions to a level of management not involved in the initial disciplinary hearing, but they must present their appeal with the grounds to the Chair of the disciplinary panel within 14 days. Their case will be heard by two managers more senior to the Chair of the original panel.

The Capability Procedure

Poor performance or conduct can be the result of either incompetence or physical or mental disability, so this process was designed to deal with concerns resulting from lack of capability. Such concerns include inappropriate practice due to lack of knowledge or failure to update it, inability to work in a team, illnesses, stress or addictions. Where possible, these issues should be resolved at a local level and this may include retraining, supervised practice, referral to healthcare services, counselling or mentoring. If this proves unsuccessful, the matter should be referred to the PPA and a capability panel.

The process follows the formal route above in that the Case Investigator will use the same methods to produce a report for the Case Manager and the practitioner has a similar right of response. The Case Manager again has to decide whether there is a case for restriction or exclusion and must take advice from the PPA. Having discussed the case with the Medical and HR Directors, the Case Manager can decide to try local resolution again before any further action but if the practitioners' practice is too fundamentally flawed to be changed, he will be referred for a panel hearing.

The Case Manager must give the practitioner 20 days' notice of the capability hearing and provide the time, date and place, allegations, rights of representation and any documentary evidence. The HCP can be accompanied by a friend or a representative from their Union or indemnity provider, but they cannot act in a legal capacity unless the HCP is facing dismissal. There must be an exchange of any evidence that each side intend to use at the hearing no more than 10 days before the hearing. The list of witnesses for each side must be presented no less than 2 days in advance. The panel consists of three people—two Trust Directors and an independent HCP in the same specialty as the accused. It is usually chaired by the Chief Executive of the Board and there are advisers from HR and another clinician in the same speciality with no connection to the case to advise on the expected level of competence for the grade of the HCP in question. The hearing follows the same procedure as the disciplinary hearing above, and once the Panel decides on any disciplinary action, their decision must be confirmed in writing within 5 days, stating the reasons for the decision and the rights of appeal. The Panel can make the following decisions:

1. No action required.

2. **Oral agreement**—there must be a significant improvement in performance within a specified timescale and this stays on the personal file for 6 months.

3. **Written warning**—there must be a significant improvement in performance within a specified timescale and this stays on the record for a year.

4. **Final written warning**—there must be a significant improvement in performance within a specified timescale, but this is for more than serious performance issues and also stays on the file for a year.

5. **Termination of contract**.

Appeals Against Capability Sanctions

HCPs can appeal against any action, but this must be sent to the Director of Human Resources within 25 days. All NHS organisations must have an internal policy for appeals to be heard by an Appeals panel, which also has three members, one of which must be independent of the Trust and taken from a pool of specially trained NHS managers. The Panel can uphold or vary the decision or require the case to be reheard and their decision must be sent to the Trust and the appellant within five working days.

Restriction and Exclusion

If there are serious concerns about an HCPs conduct, the Trust may place temporary restrictions on them, up to and including exclusion or suspension. Suspension is the most immediate, humiliating and professionally damaging consequence of any allegation made against an HCP even though it is intended to be 'neutral act' to protect interests of patients, other staff or the practitioner and/or to assist the investigative process, not a sanction. Where exclusion is the only solution, it should be done for as short a time as possible and the PPA should be notified. The practitioner must be given the opportunity to answer the allegations and provide reasons why he should not be excluded, but if the Trust decides to go ahead, the exclusion must only be for 4 weeks in the first instance and confirmed in writing. Allegations leading to suspension should be substantiated within 14 days and the suspension should be reviewed every 2 weeks, with the practitioner being informed of the outcome. The investigation should be completed within 3 months or reasons given to Trust Board. Suspension applies to all grades of HCP and the only recourse is an industrial tribunal—there is no legal remedy, as it is not regarded in law as very damaging because the HCP is on full pay throughout.

Premature Retirement

Under Health Circular *HSG(95)25*, NHS Trusts can retire a doctor prematurely on the grounds of the 'efficiency of the service'. This procedure applies to doctors whose performance has shown a consistent decline to an unacceptable level and is considered unlikely to improve despite appropriate remedial action. It may be preceded by a period of 'gardening leave', where the doctor is given leave on full pay for a period usually not exceeding 6 months. It is used for sick doctors, e.g. those with alcohol use disorder or dementia and it theoretically allows time for the doctor to 'recover from illness' but he is rarely reinstated.

Employment Tribunals

- These provide a limited remedy for racial and sexual discrimination and unfair dismissal, including 'constructive dismissal'. This is behaviour of the employer such that the employee is entitled to terminate his employment and consider himself dismissed, e.g. being instructed to work in a different hospital from that to which he is contracted.
- The HCP must have been employed by the Trust for at least 2 years and must make his application within 3 months of the date of dismissal.
- The Trust must show that the dismissal was fair, i.e. the burden of proof is on the Trust and for this to be true, the dismissal must be based on:
  1. capability or qualification
  2. misconduct
  3. restriction imposed by statute, e.g. loss of registration
  4. redundancy
  5. some other substantial reason.

- The fundamental inadequacy of an employment tribunal is that if the HCP is found to have been unfairly dismissed, he may not *necessarily* get his job back as the tribunal cannot enforce the order for reinstatement. It can only 'fine' the employer by making them pay an additional award to the employee on top of the normal compensation, which is a basic award of years of service (up to a maximum of 20) multiplied by their weekly wage.

DISCIPLINARY PROCEDURES IN GENERAL PRACTICE

NHS England has overall responsibility for commissioning primary care services, but this has been increasingly delegated to the Clinical Commissioning Groups (CCGs). Each NHS-commissioned general practice must hold an NHS GP contract, which sets out the mandatory provisions and services as well as optional ones and includes the geographical or population area, key policies and the requirement to maintain a patient list. There is a wide range of contracts available to GPs, including partners, salaried GPs and locums, but to train and work as a GP in the United Kingdom, all GPs must be on one of the primary medical performers lists, which are managed by primary care organisations (PCOs). All general practices must have their own formal disciplinary procedure and it should follow the *ACAS Code of Practice on Discipline and Grievance*. This can be used to sanction or even remove a GP from the practice and is primarily used for locums and salaried doctors. PCOs in England and Wales and Health Boards in Scotland also have the power to suspend GPs on their performers list and any GP facing suspension proceedings should contact their medical defence organisation. There is no right of appeal against suspension, but the PCO must give the doctor notice of the allegations against him, the likely action that it will take and provide the GP with the opportunity to have an oral hearing. The suspension should not last more than 6 months unless it has been imposed pending the outcome of investigations by the GMC or the police.

DEALING WITH A COLLEAGUE WHO IS UNDERPERFORMING

1. Wherever possible, discuss your concerns with your colleague directly and preferably face-to-face, although a letter or telephone call may be easier.
2. If this is not feasible, ask another HCP who is known to be a close friend of the person concerned to speak to him, as this may make him less defensive and more likely to seek help.

3. If the problem appears to be related to his health and the safety of patients may be at risk, try to contact his GP.
4. If the problem is not health related, you can voice your concerns to his immediate senior, the Local Medical Committee (for GPs), the Clinical or Medical Director (for Consultants), the Director of Nursing or the Chief Executive of the Trust.
5. If local resolution is either inappropriate or unsatisfactory, the problem is obviously serious or the HCP has committed a criminal offence, you should contact the NMC or the GMC as appropriate
6. In all cases, you must inform the person concerned of your actions but limit any information given to those who must know in order to investigate the matter further or you may be vulnerable to an action for slander or libel.
7. Make sure that your facts are accurate and verifiable but note that any clinical records used should not identify the patient unless it is unavoidable.
8. Try to be objective and make any potential conflict of interest known, e.g. a preexisting disagreement with the person concerned.
9. Note that both the GMC and the NMC have stated that HCPs have an 'ethical responsibility to act where they believe a colleague's conduct, performance or health is a threat to patients' and if they ignore this responsibility, they put themselves at risk of action by their disciplinary body.
10. Under the *Public Interest Disclosure Act 1998*, you cannot be victimised, subjected to a detriment, dismissed or made redundant after making a 'protected disclosure', i.e. only to the relevant bodies. The disclosure must concern matters of public interest such as criminal offences or health and safety concerns and be made in good faith, so it cannot be anonymous. If the concerns are not acted upon or if you believe that you are being victimised, then you can legitimately take your concerns externally, e.g. to the police, media or the DoH. However, this must be considered 'reasonable' by any subsequent tribunal and must not breach patient confidentiality. If you are sacked, you can apply for an interim order to keep your job before appearing before a tribunal and if you are then found to have been unfairly dismissed, you will be eligible for unlimited compensation.

SUMMARY

This chapter outlines the structure and function of the three main regulatory bodies—the General Medical Council, the Nursing and Midwifery Council and the Health and Care Professions Council. It discusses their different roles before going into more detail about the various disciplinary procedures held by the regulatory bodies, hospitals and within general practices. It provides helpful advice about dealing with concerns, appearing before a disciplinary hearing, what information must be provided by law and the rights of appeal.

NOTES

1. *The Shipman inquiry fifth report, safeguarding patients, lessons from the past—proposals for the future*: Cm 6394 December 2004.
2. See www.gmc-uk.org/ethical-guidance/ethical-guidance-for-doctors.
3. See www.nmc.org.uk/globalassets/sitedocuments/nmc-publications/nmc-code.pdf.

FURTHER READING

Department of Health. *Maintaining high professional standards in the modern NHS: a framework for the initial handling of concerns about doctors and dentists in the NHS*. London: DoH; 2003.

USEFUL WEBSITES

General Medical Council: www.gmc-uk.org
Nursing and Midwifery Council: www.nmc.org.uk
Health Care and Professions Council: www.hcpc-uk.org

CHAPTER 11

Death and the Healthcare Professional

INTRODUCTION

As will be discussed in Chapter 12, there is no statutory definition of death in the United Kingdom and the diagnosis of death remains a matter of clinical judgement.[1] When a person is thought to have died, a healthcare professional (HCP) will be called to 'certify the body'. However, since only a doctor can issue a death certificate and then only under very limited circumstances, it is more accurate to describe the process as 'confirming life extinct'. If that death has occurred outside the hospital, the HCP may also be asked for an estimation of the time of death and whether he believes that there are any suspicious circumstances e.g. a potential murder or suicide. This often causes some concern so this chapter will cover the procedures involved. It will then discuss the role, courts and verdicts of the coroner and the procurator fiscal (PF).

CONFIRMATION OF DEATH

In the past, doctors were always called to confirm death, but they have **no legal obligation** to:
1. confirm death
2. view the dead body
3. report the fact of a death, although they must report the **cause** of death if they attended the deceased during the final illness.

In English law, **any** competent adult can confirm death and there have been significant changes in who is allowed to confirm death in the wake of the COVID-19 pandemic. There are now arrangements in place for verification of death to be performed by a wider range of health and social care workers, especially in residential and care homes and where home carers are employed. In areas where such workers still need support, the British Medical Association (BMA) and the Royal College of General Practitioners (RCGP) have produced a protocol for remote assistance in verifying death.[2] Suspicious deaths must still be reported to the police and unexpected deaths should be reported to the local coroner so that the cause of death can be established.

DEATHS OUT OF HOSPITAL
On Arrival

- If the death is expected, confirm death (see later) and inform those in attendance that they can contact the undertaker. If you are able to sign the Medical Certificate of Cause of Death (MCCD) (see later), then do so as this enables the family to register the death.
- If the death is unexpected but there are no suspicious circumstances, confirm death and inform the coroner, either through the coroner's officer or the police. Do *not* sign an MCCD until agreed by the coroner. Tell those in attendance that the coroner's officer will either arrange for the body to be removed or allow them to call the undertaker.
- If the death is unexpected and it appears that there may be suspicious circumstances, call the police. If they are already present, talk to the officer in charge, as you must not disturb or contaminate any potential evidence during your examination. It may have to be much more limited and only done once the scene has been photographed. You will also be shown the route to follow when approaching and leaving the body.

  Remember that the police can investigate any scene that they consider suspicious, but if you state that you believe that the cause of death was not natural, then they must investigate the scene further. .

Take a History

This may come from the police and/or the relatives. Try to ascertain:

- When and where the person was last seen or heard and by whom. This will give you clues when trying to estimate how long the person has been dead. It may also be useful in deciding whewther or not there are suspicious circumstances e.g. the relative who claims to have seen the person the day before when life has obviously been extinct for much longer
- How and where the body was discovered and by whom. The body should not have been moved but this is not always the case, particularly if attempts have been made at resuscitation by the relatives or ambulance personnel
- Any relevant past medical or surgical history. This may help in establishing the cause of death although this is **not** your role, other than giving an opinion as to whether it was natural or not.

Note the Surroundings

Detailed crime scene investigation is the role of the police, but it is useful to note the following:

- Signs of forced entry, other than those caused by the police who have a power of entry if they consider that lives may be at risk
- Medication, including empty bottles
- Drug paraphernalia e.g. 'crack' pipes, syringes
- Signs of alcohol abuse e.g. empty cans and bottles
- Signs of neglect
- The temperature of the room (see later)
- The dates of any newspapers or letters.

Examine the Body

As stated, your examination may be limited to observation only and if so, you should note:

- Any obvious injuries, particularly potentially lethal wounds, defence injuries or signs of previous self-harm. Describe them accurately in your notes (see Chapter 3)
- Any signs of struggle
- The site and position of the body
- The condition and position of any clothing
- Any blood or vomit around the mouth and nose
- Signs of post mortem hypostasis (see later)
- Potential instruments of murder or suicide e.g. a ligature around the neck
- Any stigmata of chronic disease e.g. spider naevi in liver disease

- Any obvious scars, particularly surgical ones.

If you are allowed to touch the body, then also check:

- The temperature of the body (see later)
- Any movement in the small and large joints (see later)
- If you can turn the body over, check for any hidden injuries, marks or scars.

Confirm Death

Death in situations other than those described in Chapter 12 is usually confirmed by noting the absence of the carotid pulse, breath and heart sounds. If the person has only recently died, then you must listen to the chest for several minutes as there are many conditions that may mimic death e.g. hypothermia, coma and drug overdoses. It is distressing to note that in the home situation, the person has often been dead for weeks to months and there is rarely any doubt that the person is dead, but mistakes have been made and you must be absolutely certain that life is extinct before sending the body to the mortuary.

State the Time of Death

The legal date and time of death is that which you state on completion of your examination of the body, even if you believe that the person actually died months earlier.

Talk to the Relatives

If there are relatives present, it is important to talk to them. Be sympathetic and if there are no suspicious circumstances, reassure them that there was nothing else that could have been done to save their relative. It is vital to try to help them with the guilt that they inevitably feel and even if you think that earlier medical intervention might have changed the outcome, there is **nothing** to be gained from expressing this belief. If possible, tell them that you think that their relative did not suffer but do not try to guess at the cause of death unless you are in a position to issue a certificate (see later). Warn them if you think that post mortem will be necessary but reassure them that it should not interfere with their funeral arrangements unless there is any suspicion that the cause of death was not natural. Ask them if they have any further questions before leaving but if you do not know the answer, say so.

DEATHS IN HOSPITAL

Confirming death in hospital is much simpler as there are rarely suspicious circumstances, although this may occur, such as when a psychiatric patient successfully commits suicide. You may be asked to confirm death in the back of the ambulance so the patient can be taken directly to the mortuary, but this should never be done if there are relatives present unless there is no hope of resuscitation, e.g. a person decapitated in a road accident. Even when confirming death in a ward patient, you should still take a history as mentioned earlier and also refer to the hospital notes. You must examine the body thoroughly prior to confirming death, as a death in hospital does not necessarily equate to a death from natural causes.

ESTIMATION OF TIME OF DEATH

This is a subject of much debate and while the following may give clues towards the likely time of death, none are 100% accurate and you should not be too dogmatic in your estimate. There are many good books on the subject (see the Further reading list), so the following provides an outline only.

Rigor Mortis

After death, the muscle glycogen stores start to deplete and ATP (adenosine triphosphate) can no longer be resynthesised from adenosine diphosphate (ADP). This results in a sustained contraction in all the muscles and subsequent stiffness, known as rigor mortis. The effects are most pronounced in the small muscles initially, so the jaw, finger and toe joints are affected first. As the process continues, the larger joints such as the hips, knees and elbows become affected. As time progresses, the muscles then start to deteriorate, the contracture decreases and the body becomes flaccid again. The onset of rigor mortis is very variable and is affected by factors such as the ambient temperature—it occurs earlier with higher temperatures—and the level of initial glycogen stores, so it starts sooner if the person was very active prior to death e.g. struggling or fitting. Generally, the duration of rigor mortis follows the pattern shown later but its use in determining the time of death is limited by the variation (Table 11.1).

Cadaveric spasm is an extreme variant that occurs immediately after death. The mechanism is not understood but it is more common in people who have suffered a severe 'fight or flight' reaction just prior to death e.g. soldiers. Fire victims may be found in a 'pugilistic attitude', where their stance suggests that they are about to punch someone. This is caused by heat contractures within the flexor muscles.

TABLE 11.1
Pattern of Rigor Mortis

Time of Death (hours)	Pattern
<3	Body is warm and flaccid
3–6	The small muscles contract and the jaw, toe and finger joints stiffen
6–12	The larger muscles contract and the hip, knee and elbow joints stiffen
12–18	Rigor mortis is complete
18–36	The muscles start to deteriorate and the small, then large joints become mobile
>36	Body is cold and flaccid

TABLE 11.2
Relevance of Colour of Lividity

Colour	Caused by	Likely Cause of Death
Cherry red	Carboxyhaemo-globin	Carbon monoxide poisoning
Pink	Undissociated oxyhaemoglobin	Hypothermia
Dark red	Oxygenated blood	Cyanide poisoning
Grey-brown	Methaemoglobi-naemia	Ethylene glycol poisoning (antifreeze)

Post Mortem Hypostasis

This is also known as lividity and occurs as a result of gravitational pooling of blood. It looks similar to bruising and is seen in dependent areas of the body although pressure points are paler due to sparing. It also has a very variable onset but usually starts about an hour after death and becomes complete after 6 to 12 hours. It then becomes 'fixed' and remains unchanged until putrefaction occurs. The variability in onset means that it cannot be accurately used to assess time of death but if it is seen in nondependent areas, it suggests that the body was moved after death. It may be very faint if the death was preceded by massive haemorrhage. The normal colour is blue/red but different colours may give an idea of the cause of death (Table 11.2).

Temperature

Traditional teaching states that the body temperature declines at a rate of 0.9°C per hour after death, but this is inaccurate as body cooling occurs in a sigmoid fashion, not linear, and it varies with many different factors such as:

- Clothing
- Ambient temperature, humidity and air movement
- Body temperature immediately before death, e.g. fever or hypothermia
- Body fat or oedema, which acts as an insulator
- Immersion.

A rectal thermometer is more likely to give an accurate reading than a surface one, but this may interfere with the forensic evidence so it should not be done at the scene. Any comments regarding the temperature of the body are best limited to whether the body feels cold or warm to the touch.

Decomposition

Putrefaction is the process by which the body disintegrates tissue. It also has a very variable time of onset and depends on many factors such as:

- Ambient temperature—the hotter the surroundings, the quicker the onset
- Body fat or oedema, which hastens putrefaction
- Burial or immersion in water, which delays the changes.

It usually starts on the third day after death as a greenish discolouration of the right iliac fossa over the caecum. This spreads and reaches the face by about 7 days when the skin starts to blister and erode. Gas formation starts in the softer tissues around the neck, abdomen and genitals and involves the whole body by the end of the second week. In warm, humid surroundings, the body fat may be converted to a waxy substance called 'adipocere', which may persist for years. If the body is in warm, dry surroundings, it can mummify and become brown and leathery.

Other Methods

Other methods of determining the time of death include:

- Biochemical changes in the blood, urine and cerebrospinal fluid
- Eye changes—segmentation in the retinal blood vessels; corneal opacity and dark marks on the sclera ('taches noires sclerotiques')
- Entomology—the presence or absence of different types of maggots and other parasites
- Botany—growth of different types of plants through interred or concealed bodies.

DEATH CERTIFICATION IN ENGLAND AND WALES

Certification of death must be done accurately and promptly, as it provides legal evidence of the fact and cause of death. This allows the death to be registered so the family can make arrangements to dispose of the body and the data can be used for mortality statistics. About 75% of deaths in the United Kingdom are certified by a doctor and the remainder by the coroner. There are three types of certificates:

1. **Stillbirth Certificate** (>24 weeks gestation)—this is completed by the doctor or midwife present at the birth and the death must be registered within 42 days in England, 21 days in Scotland and a year in Northern Ireland.
2. **Neonatal Death Certificate** (any death up to 28 days of age)—the death must be registered within 8 days in Scotland and 5 days in the rest of the United Kingdom.
3. **Medical Certificate of Cause of Death (MCCD)**— also known as the 'death certificate' (all other deaths—see Figs 11.1 and 11.2).

Under Section 22 of the *Births and Deaths Registration Act 1953*, a doctor who has attended the deceased during his last illness has a statutory duty to sign the MCCD, stating the cause of death to the 'best of his knowledge and belief' **unless** the death is one that should be reported to the coroner. As shown in Fig. 11.1, the form is divided into three parts:

1. The left side is a counterfoil, which remains in the book and must be completed at the same time as the certificate, as a record of the information provided.
2. The right side is a 'Notice to Informant', which confirms that the certificate has been issued to the relatives or other authorised persons. Note that this part is absent on the forms used in Northern Ireland and Scotland introduced a new MCCD in 2015, which eliminates the need for doctors to complete a separate cremation form (see later).
3. The centre part is the actual certificate. This must be taken to Registrar within 5 days (8 days in Scotland).

If you are asked to complete an MCCD, you should note the following:

- You must be a registered medical practitioner (full or provisional) with a licence to practice in the United Kingdom and you must have attended the deceased during his last illness. Prior to the COVID-19 pandemic, you must also have seen the deceased either within 14 days of the death or after it, but the provisions of the *Coronavirus Act 2020* extended this to

MED A
14   000000

COUNTERFOIL

For use of Medical Practitioner,
who should complete in all cases.

Name of }
deceased }

Date of death

Place of death

Last seen alive }
by me }

Post-mortem?*   1   2   3   4
Coroner

Whether seen   a   b   c
after death*

Cause of death

I (a)

   (b)

   (c)

Employment? [ ] *Please tick where applicable*

B. Further information offered?

Signature

Date

* *Ring appropriate digit(s) and letter*

MED A
14   000000

                    Registrar to enter
                    No. of Death Entry

BIRTHS AND DEATHS REGISTRATION ACT 1953
(Form prescribed by the Registration of Births, Deaths and Marriages (Amendment) Regulations 1968)
MEDICAL CERTIFICATE OF CAUSE OF DEATH
For use only by a registered Medical Practitioner WHO HAS BEEN IN ATTENDANCE during the deceased's last illness,
and to be delivered by him forthwith to the Registrar of Births and Deaths

Name of deceased
Date of death as stared to me .... day of .... 19...... Age as stated to me ....
Place of death .... day of .... 19......
Last seen alive by me .... day of .... 19......

Please ring
appropriate
digit(s) and letter

a Seen after death by me
b Seen after death by **another medical practitioner**
   but not by me
c Not seen after death by a medical practitioner

CAUSE OF DEATH
*The condition thought to be the 'Underlying Cause of Death' should
appear in the lowest completed line of Part I*

*These particulars not to be
entered in death register*

Approximate interval
between onset and death

I (a) Disease or condition directly
      leading to death **
   (b) Other disease or condition, if any,
      leading to I (a)
   (c) Other disease or condition, if any,
      leading to (b).

II Other significant conditions
    CONTRIBUTING TO THE DEATH but
    not related to the disease or condition
    causing it.

The death might have been due to or contributed to by the employment followed at some time by the deceased. [ ] Please tick where applicable

†This does not mean the mode of dying, such as heart failure, asphyxia, asthenia, etc. It means the disease, injury, or complication which caused death

**I hereby certify that I was in medical attendance during
the above named deceased's last illness, and that the
particulars and cause of death above written are true
to the best of my knowledge and belief**

Qualifications as registered }
by General Medical Council }

Signature
Residence .... Date

For death in hospital: Please give the name of the consultant responsible for the above-named as a patient ....

MED A
14   000000

(Form prescribed by the Registration of Births,
Deaths and Marriages Regulations 1968)

NOTICE TO INFORMANT

I hereby give notice that I have this day signed a
medical certificate of cause of death of

Signature ....
    Date ....
This notice is to be delivered by the informant to the
registrar of births and deaths for the sub-district in
which the death occurred.

The certifying medical practitioner must give this
notice to the person who is qualified and liable to act
as informant for the registration of death (see list
overleaf).

DUTIES OF INFORMANT

Failure to deliver this notice to the registrar renders
the informant liable to prosecution. The death cannot be
registered until the medical certificate has reached the
registrar.

When the death is registered the informant must be
prepared to give to the registrar the following particulars
relating to the deceased:

1. The date and place of death

2. The full name and surname (and the maiden
    surname if the deceased was a woman who had
    married).

3. The date and place of birth.

4. The occupation (and if the deceased was a married
    woman or a widow the name and occupation of her
    husband)

5. The usual address.

6. Whether the deceased was in receipt of a pension
    or allowance from public funds.

7. If the deceased was married, the date of birth of the
    surviving widow or widower.

**THE DECEASED'S MEDICAL CARD SHOULD BE
DELIVERED TO THE REGISTRAR**

FIG. 11.1 Medical Certificate of Cause of Death (MCCD)—front of the form.

PERSONS QUALIFIED AND LIABLE TO ACT AS INFORMANTS

The following persons are designated by the Births and Deaths Registration Act 1953 as qualified to give information concerning a death:–

(1) A relative of the deceased, present at the death.

(2) A relative of the deceased, in attendance during the last illness.

(3) A relative of the deceased, residing or being in the sub-district where the death occurred.

(4) A person present at the death.

(5) The occupier* if he knew of the happening of the death.

(6) Any inmate if he knew of the happening of the death.

(7) The person causing the disposal of the body.

DEATHS IN HOUSES OR DEAD BODIES FOUND

(1) Any relative of the deceased having knowledge of any of the particulars required to be registered.

(2) Any person present at the death.

(3) Any person who found the body.

(4) Any person in charge of the body.

(5) The person causing the disposal of the body.

* "Occupier" in relation to a public institution includes the governor, keeper, matron, superintendent, or other chief resident officer.

Complete where applicable

A

I have reported this death to the Coroner for further action.

Initials of certifying medical practitioner.

The Coroner needs to consider all cases where:
The death might have been due to or contributed to by a violent or unnatural cause (including an accident);

or   the cause of death cannot be identified:

or   the death might have been due to or contributed to by drugs, medicine, abortion or poison:

B

I may be in a position later to give, on application by the Registrar General, additional information as to the cause of death for the purpose or more precise statistical classification.

Initials of certifying medical practitioner.

or   there is reason to believe that the death occurred during an operation or under or prior to complete recovery from an operation or an anaesthetic:

or   the death might have been due to or contributed to by the employment followed at some time by the deceased.

LIST OF SOME OF THE CATEGORIES OF DEATH WHICH MAY BE OF INDUSTRIAL ORIGIN

MALIGNANT DISEASES

Causes include:

(a) Skin
–radiation and sunlight
–pitch tar
–mineral oils

(b) Nasal
–wood or leather work
–nickel

(c) Lungs
–asbestos
–nickel
–radiation

(d) Pleura
–asbestos

(e) Urinary Tract
–benzidine
–dyestuff
–chemicals in rubber

(f) Liver
–PVC manufacture

(g) Bone
–radiation

(h) Lymphatics and haematopoietic
–radiation
–benzene

POISONING

(a) Metals
e.g. arsenics, cadmium, lead

(b) Chemicals
e.g. chlorine, benzene

(c) Solvents
e.g. trichlorethylene

INFECTIOUS DISEASES

Causes include:

(a) Anthrax
imported bone, bonemeal, hide or fur

(b) Brucellosis
farming or veterinary contact at work

(c) Tuberculosis

(d) Leptospirosis
farming, sewer or under-ground workers

(e) Tetanus
farming or gardening

(f) Rabies
animal handling

(g) Viral hepatitis
contact at work

BRONCHIAL ASTHMA AND PNEUMONITIS

(a) Occupational asthma
sensitising agent at work

(b) Allergic Alveolitis
farming

PNEUMOCONIOSIS

mining and quarrying
potteries
asbestos

NOTE:–The Practitioner, on signing the certificate, should complete, sign and date the Notice to the Informant, which should be detached and handed to the Informant.The Practitioner should then, without delay, deliver the certificate itself to the Registrar of Births and Deaths for the sub-district in which the death occurred. Envelopes for enclosing the certificates are supplied by the Registrar.

FIG. 11.2 Medical Certificate of Cause of Death (MCCD) – back of the form.

28 days, changed 'attending' to 'any' doctor and included video link as an acceptable method of 'seeing' the (live) patient. If you or another doctor have seen him in the preceding 28 days, then there is no **legal** requirement for you to see the body after death before you complete the MCCD, but it is good practice to do so. If these conditions have not been met but you remain satisfied about the likely cause of death, you can still complete an MCCD, but you must clearly state that the deceased was not seen within 28 days of death or after it and inform the coroner. You will then be asked to explain to the coroner why you are so certain of the cause of death so that he can make a determination. The coroner can then either issue a Form 100A sanctioning the MCCD or order a post mortem examination (see later).

- MCCDs should be completed legibly, honestly, accurately and promptly.
- The most important part of the MCCD is the actual cause of death, which is divided into Parts I and II:
  - Part I should indicate the disease or condition directly leading to the death and it is further subdivided into parts a, b and c to allow for more than one condition or complication.
  - Part II should list any contributing diseases not directly related to the condition causing the death, e.g. Part I might be ischaemic heart disease and Part II, diabetes or smoking.
- Note that COVID-19 is an acceptable direct or underlying cause of death, but it does not need to be referred to the coroner even though it is a notifiable disease under *Health Protection (Notification) Regulations 2010*.
- Do not record the mode of death and never give it as the cause of death, e.g. heart failure or cardiac arrest.
- Never use abbreviations as this can lead to ambiguity, e.g. M.S. may mean mitral stenosis, multiple sclerosis or Marfan syndrome.
- You can now give 'old age' or 'natural causes' as a cause of death but only if you cannot give a more specific cause and the deceased was >80 years.
- Do not withhold sensitive information in deference to the relatives.
- Refer to the notes and directions contained in the book of certificates as these are a useful source of help and advice. The books are held in either the GP surgery or the Bereavement Office at the hospital.
- If you are in hospital, you must give the name of the Consultant in charge of the patient. This is because the Registrar may require further information in the future and junior staff change frequently.

- If you issue a certificate in a case that you wish to report to the coroner, initial box A (Fig. 11.2) on the back of the certificate. This will alert the Registrar, but you will also need to talk to the coroner directly. Do not complete it if you have discussed the case with the coroner's office already and they have said that a referral is not necessary.
- If you wish to wait for the results of tests prior to categorising the death, initial box B (Fig. 11.2) on the back of the form. There is also a space on the front of the form to indicate that the results of a post mortem may be available later.
- If in doubt, discuss the case with the coroner's officer.

The introduction of the *Notification of Deaths Regulations 2019* means that doctors now have a **statutory** duty to notify the coroner where there is reasonable cause to believe that the death was **due** to any of the factors shown in Box 11.1.

The coroner must be informed 'as soon as is reasonably practical' and the reporting doctor must provide the following information:

1. Their own full contact details
2. The full name, date of birth, sex, address and occupation of the deceased.

BOX 11.1
Deaths That Should Be Reported to the Coroner

- Poisoning, including acute alcohol intoxication
- Exposure to a toxic substance
- Use of a prescribed, controlled or over-the-counter drug or psychoactive substance. This includes drug errors
- The cause of death is unknown even if the doctor was in regular attendance
- The deceased was not attended by a doctor during his last illness
- The deceased was not seen by a doctor either after death or within the 28 days before death
- Violence, trauma or injury
- Medical treatment or procedure, whether the death occurred as a direct or indirect result, e.g. following surgery or infection
- Accidental deaths
- Deaths that may have been due to neglect—either by self or others
- Deaths that may have been caused by industrial disease or related to employment
- Deaths following an abortion
- Suicides and self-harm
- Deaths that occurred during an operation or before recovery from the anaesthetic
- Deaths in custody

3. The name and address of the next of kin or person with parental responsibility (if the deceased was a child) or the person or local authority that will be responsible for the disposal of the body
4. The reason why the death has been referred to the coroner
5. The place, date and time of death
6. The name of any Consultant or GP who attended the deceased within the last 14 days
7. Any other relevant information.

If the deceased died from natural causes, the following may occur:

1. There are no reasons to report the death to the coroner, so the doctor completes the MCCD unless a post mortem is requested for clinical interest. This is done to establish the extent of the disease, not the cause of death although a study in 2001 showed that in over 60% cases that had a post mortem for this purpose, the predicted cause of death was wrong.[3]
2. The death was reported but a natural cause can be established without a post mortem and the coroner issues a Form 100 A to the Registrar. This informs him that death was due to natural causes and he advises the doctor to complete the MCCD.
3. A post mortem examination is deemed necessary but reveals a natural cause of death. The coroner issues a Form 100B to the Registrar, informing him of the cause of death and that no further action is required.

Once the Registrar receives either the MCCD or Form 100B, he registers the death and issues a disposal certificate. If the deceased died of unnatural causes, then an inquest must be held.

MEDICAL EXAMINERS

The new system of medical examiners (MEs) was first proposed following the publication of the third report of the Shipman inquiry.[4] This said that there should be an effective crosscheck when the treating doctor completed the MCCD, purporting to also know the cause of death to 'not only deter a doctor such as Shipman but also to deter any doctor who might be tempted to conceal activity less serious than murder, such as an error or neglect by himself or a colleague'. The *Coroners and Justice Act 2009* subsequently set out a new system of death certification whereby all deaths not referred to the coroner would be scrutinised by independent MEs for both burials and cremations and all acute Trusts in England and Health Boards in Wales were asked to set up ME offices. Their role is to[5]:

- agree the proposed cause of death and the overall accuracy of the MCCD with the completing doctor
- discuss the cause of death with the next of kin/informant and establish if they have questions or any concerns with the care before death
- act as a medical advice resource for the local coroner
- prepare the selection of cases for further review under local mortality arrangements.

The ME offices are currently used to oversee the certification of local deaths, but it is intended that the role will be made statutory and extended to all noncoronial deaths, wherever they occur. MEs are senior doctors with additional legal training that work on a contractual basis and they are supported by ME officers. The purpose of the ME system is to[5]:

- provide greater safeguards for the public by ensuring proper scrutiny of all noncoronial deaths
- ensure the appropriate direction of deaths to the coroner
- provide a better service for the bereaved and an opportunity for them to raise any concerns to a doctor not involved in the care of the deceased
- improve the quality of death certification
- improve the quality of mortality data.

THE CORONER SYSTEM

Coroners date from 1194, but the office has evolved from a predominantly fiscal role in protecting the royal revenues to that of an independent judicial officer responsible for the investigation of all unnatural deaths occurring within his district. There are 98 coroners in England and Wales covering 109 coroner's areas and the caseloads vary. Currently, coroners can be medically or legally qualified (often both) but following the introduction of the *Coroners and Justice Act 2009*, all future coroners must be legally qualified. This act also created the new role of Chief Coroner and changed the hierarchy of coroners to senior coroners, area coroners and assistant coroners. The role of the Chief Coroner is to provide judicial oversight of the coroner system, so he must be a senior judge appointed by the Lord Chief Justice. Coroners are appointed by the local authority with the consent of the Lord Chancellor and the Chief Coroner, but can only be removed by the Lord Chancellor. They are not allowed to determine criminal liability following the enactment of the *Criminal Law Act 1977*, so the last inquest to name the accused was that of Sandra Rivett, nanny to Lord Lucan, where the jury returned a verdict naming Lord Lucan as her murderer.

The Role of the Coroner

Under Section 5 of the *Coroners and Justice Act 2009*, the role of the coroner is to undertake an investigation into the causes and circumstances of a death to determine:

- Who died
- When they died
- Where they died
- How they died

The jurisdiction of the coroner relates to the presence of the body in his district, irrespective of where the person actually died so it includes people who have died abroad but have been returned home. Following the enactment of the *Coroners (Investigations) Regulations 2013*, coroners can now also conduct inquests in other districts if it is in the best interests of the bereaved family.

The 2009 Act means that the coroner can now perform an investigation before deciding if it is necessary to hold an inquest, but if the coroner does decide to hold an inquest, he must do so within 6 months of becoming aware of the death or 'as soon as reasonably practicable'. The coroner has a duty under Section 1 of the Act to investigate a death if it occurred in his area and there is reasonable cause to suspect that the death:

1. Was violent or unnatural
2. Remains of unknown cause despite a post mortem
3. Occurred in custody or state detention, so his remit has been extended to include other parts of the detention estate such as mental health hospitals and immigration removal centres.

The coroner usually sits alone but a jury of 7 to 11 members joins him for:

1. Violent, unknown cause or unnatural deaths in custody or state detention or as a result of an act or omission by a police officer in the purported execution of his duty. Juries are no longer necessary for natural deaths in custody.
2. Industrial deaths, including accidents, poisoning and diseases, e.g. asbestosis.
3. Deaths where the coroner thinks there is 'sufficient cause' to have a jury, e.g. major incidents such as train crashes.

Where someone has been charged with causing the death, the inquest will be adjourned until after the trial, but the death will be registered. The coroner may give permission for the body to be cremated or buried in the interim if this would not result in loss of valuable evidence.

Appearing at an Inquest

The conduct of an inquest is governed by the *Coroners and Justice Act 2009* and it is inquisitorial in nature, unlike the adversarial approach of the remainder of the British legal systems (see Chapter 1). All information is shared unless there is a restriction to disclosure prior to the inquest and the coroner decides which witnesses should be called. Hearings are public, unless there is an issue of national security and anyone can offer to give evidence or inform the coroner that they believe that a particular witness should be called. As for any other court, the coroner can compel a witness to attend upon penalty of a fine or even imprisonment, but he can now accept a written statement if there are compelling reasons why the witness cannot attend and the evidence is unlikely to be contested.

The degree of formality varies but it can be very intimidating, particularly if the family of the deceased is present, and you must dress smartly. As for the other courts, you will be expected to have brought any relevant notes, investigations and X-rays. Evidence is given under oath or affirmation and you should follow the advice given in Chapter 2. You will initially be examined by the coroner and this is usually quite neutral, merely seeking to establish the facts of the case. Hearsay evidence is allowed and you may be asked to comment on the medical notes made by others. Although many coroners are also medically qualified, use layman's terms wherever possible so that the family can understand. You may then be questioned by any 'interested persons' as defined in Section 47 of the 2009 Act—either in person or through a legal representative. Please see Box 11.2.

Questions must be sensible and the coroner can insist that you answer all relevant questions unless it would result in self-incrimination of a criminal act. This questioning can be very difficult, particularly if there is a suggestion of negligence by yourself or your colleagues and you must try to remain calm and composed. Remember that the role of the inquest is solely to establish the identity of the deceased and how, when and where he died. It must not infer either criminal or civil liability on any named person although both types of proceedings may follow an inquest. You are also entitled to have legal representation and if you are concerned that your conduct may be called into question, then it is wise to have a legal adviser present. Note that legal aid is not available for inquests unless there are exceptional circumstances.

The term 'verdict' has now been replaced by 'conclusion' and the standard of proof is the civil standard of *balance of probabilities* for all conclusions, including suicide and unlawful killing. There are a range of *short-form* conclusions that the coroner can bring but these are the commonest:

1. Natural causes
2. Death from industrial disease

BOX 11.2
'Interested Persons'

- Parent/spouse/partner/child/sibling/grandparent or anyone acting for the deceased
- Personal representative of the deceased
- A medical examiner exercising functions in relation to the deceased
- Beneficiaries and issuers of the deceased's life insurance policy
- Anyone whose actions the coroner believes may have contributed to the death, accidentally or otherwise
- A Union representative for cases of industrial disease
- Representative of an enforcing authority
- A Chief Constable (only through a lawyer)
- Governmental officials appointed to attend the inquest
- Anyone else that the coroner decides has 'sufficient interest'

---

3. Drug or alcohol dependence and/or abuse
4. Want of attention at birth
5. Attempted or self-induced abortion
6. Stillbirth
7. Accidental death (neither the act causing the death nor the consequences were intended) or misadventure (the act was deliberate, e.g. taking prescription medication, but the consequence was not, e.g. allergic reaction)
8. Neglect, although this is usually associated with another conclusion, e.g. accidental death
9. Suicide—this must be proved to have been a voluntary act with the sole and conscious intention of killing themselves
10. Lawful killing
11. Unlawful killing—this is usually as a result of an unlawful act, e.g. murder or gross negligence manslaughter
12. Open—this means that there is insufficient evidence to decide how the deceased met his death and the case is left open in case further evidence appears.

Since 2004, the coroner may also record a *narrative* conclusion, either in addition to or instead of a short form conclusion, which records the circumstances of the death without inferring any liability.

If his investigation has revealed that something needs to be done to prevent future deaths, the coroner has a duty to send a 'Prevent Future Deaths (PFD)' report to the relevant authority but although he can recommend that action is taken, the coroner cannot dictate what that action should be. The coroner is also responsible for establishing the rightful ownership of any booty found in his district, e.g. buried treasure or the cargo of wrecked ships. This is known as establishment of 'treasure trove'.

The coroner's decisions are subject to judicial review in the High Court, but this must be requested within 3 months of the conclusion of the inquest.

DEATH CERTIFICATION IN SCOTLAND

Under the *Certification of Death (Scotland) Act 2011*, a doctor has a duty to complete an MCCD (Form 11) if he attended the deceased during the last illness, but if the attending doctor is not available any doctor who knows the cause of death may complete the certificate. The death must be registered within 8 days and since 2015, all deaths must be registered before burial or cremation can take place. The 2011 act also introduced a new system of certification, similar to the ME system called the Death Certification Review Service (DCRS), which is comprised of a Senior Medical Reviewer (SMR), a team of Medical Reviewers (MRs) and Medical Reviewers Assistants (MRAs). There are two levels of random independent reviews of MCCDs:

Level 1: a basic short review, which is completed in 10% of all deaths and should take 1 day.

Level 2: a more comprehensive review of over 1000 deaths per year and any additional reviews for cause and should take less than 3 days.

The Scottish equivalent of the coroner is the procurator fiscal (PF), who is also the public prosecutor (see Chapter 1) and there are 11 PFs in Scotland. They have a statutory duty to investigate the deaths shown in Box 11.3.

Once a death has been reported to the PF, he has legal responsibility for the body until an MCCD has been completed and given to the person registering the death. The PF will first discuss the case with the reporting doctor and if he is satisfied with the cause of death, he will advise the doctor to complete the MCCD and no further action is necessary. If he decides that it does warrant more investigation, it is done in private and may involve:

1. Interviewing the relatives or other witnesses (this is usually done on his behalf by the police). This is called 'precognition' and is not under oath.
2. Calling for a further medical report—for deaths outside hospital and the usual residence of the deceased, the forensic medical examiner (FME) may be required to externally examine the body to

> **Box 11.3**
> **Deaths That Must Be Investigated by the Procurator Fiscal**
>
> 1. Of uncertain cause
> 2. Accidental, including falls, vehicle, train or aeroplane accidents
> 3. Industrial, including accident, poisoning or disease
> 4. Following abortion or attempted abortion
> 5. Under anaesthetic
> 6. Under medical or dental care where there is reason to believe that there may have been a failure in the care or equipment, or it is likely to be the subject of an adverse incident review or where concerns have been raised
> 7. Drug-related deaths including those reportable under the Yellow Card system (see Chapter 18)
> 8. As a result of neglect, exposure or fault
> 9. Children, especially those in care or on the Child Protection Register
> 10. Perinatal death, especially sudden, unexpected, unexplained or following a concealed pregnancy
> 11. Suffocation in children, including overlaying
> 12. Poisoning
> 13. Notifiable and infectious disease
> 14. While subject to detention and/or treatment under mental health legislation
> 15. In prison or police custody
> 16. People of no fixed abode
> 17. Drowning
> 18. Fire, scalding and explosion
> 19. Possibility of suicide
> 20. Any other violent, sudden, suspicious or unexplained death

confirm death and whether there are any suspicious circumstances.

3. Ordering a post mortem, of which there are three types:
   a) *Full*—to try to establish cause of death on the 'balance of probabilities'
   b) *External examination only* ('view and grant') at the discretion of the pathologist—for probable natural deaths
   c) *'View and grant preferred'*—for cases where the relatives have a strong objection to a post mortem (this is rarely used).

If the death occurred in custody or as a result of an industrial accident or it appears to the Lord Advocate that there is public interest in the case, the PF is obliged by the *Fatal Accidents and Sudden Deaths Inquiry (Scotland) Act 2016* to hold a Fatal Accident Inquiry (FAI).

Appearing at a Fatal Accident Inquiry

The conduct of an FAI is very similar to the coroner's inquest in England (see earlier). It is inquisitorial and is held in public before the Sheriff without a jury, with the PF leading the evidence, before questions from anyone with a 'proper interest'. The PF calls the witnesses and informs any 'interested parties'. At the conclusion of the Inquiry, the Sheriff issues a determination, which is not admissible in other courts and must set out:

- Where and when the death and any accident leading to it occurred
- The cause(s) of death
- The reasonable precautions (if any) that may have prevented the death
- The defects (if any) that may have contributed to the death.
- Any other facts relevant to the circumstances of the death.

Note that the Sheriff does not have the same range of conclusions available to the coroner.

DEATH CERTIFICATION IN NORTHERN IRELAND

The coroner system in Northern Ireland is similar to that of England and Wales but the relevant statute is the *Coroner's Act (Northern Ireland) 1959* and there are some differences:

- Coroners are appointed by the Lord Chancellor and they must be barristers or solicitors. Their jurisdictions are more limited, as the death must occur or the body must be found within their district.
- In jury cases, coroners in England and Wales can accept a majority verdict but in Northern Ireland, it must be unanimous.

POST MORTEMS AND REMOVAL OF TISSUE

In deaths from natural causes, there is no legal obligation for a post mortem, but it may be requested in clinical interest to establish the extent of the disease or to look for other pathology. Under the *Human Tissue Act 2004*, authority for hospital post mortems must come from the 'person lawfully in possession of the body', which is the Trust until the body is claimed by the next of kin or the executor(s). Permission can only be given if there is no reason to believe that either the relatives or the dead person would have objected to a post mortem. Relatives can specify which organs and tissues can be removed for examination and the Human Tissue Authority (see Chapter 12) recommend that the relatives should be allowed a 'cooling off' period for 24 hours before making their final decision. If the post mortem has been authorised by the coroner, the consent of the relatives is not required. Neither the coroner nor the PF can authorise the retention of tissue for research purposes.

The *Human Tissue Act 2004* regulates the removal, storage and use of all human tissue, including cells so it also covers tissue removed at operations, e.g. following a mastectomy or a blood sample. It also created the offence of 'DNA theft', where the donor must give specific permission for DNA analysis of any tissue taken. Human tissue that has been removed or donated, e.g. bone grafts can be stored and used only for a 'designated' purpose and it is an offence to treat it in any other manner.

DISPOSAL ARRANGEMENTS

Under the *Births and Deaths Registration Act 1926*, an undertaker can only dispose of a body with either a disposal certificate from the Registrar or an *Order for Burial* (Form 101) from the coroner and he must inform the Registrar once the burial has taken place. If the relatives wish to take the body abroad for disposal or bury it at sea, they must obtain an *Out of England Order* (Form 104) from the coroner, even if the death was from natural causes. This is because there is a loss of potential medicolegal evidence. For burials at sea, they must also have a special coffin, a certificate confirming that the body is free from fever and infection and also notify the Marine Management Organisation for England and Wales or the Marine Scotland Licensing Operations Team for Scotland. There are only a very limited number of areas of the sea that can be used for sea burials, including Newhaven, Tynemouth and the Needles off the Isle of Wight.

Section 23 of the *Coroners and Justice Act 2009* gives the coroner the power to order the exhumation of a body for a post mortem to be conducted or for the purpose of possible criminal proceedings relating to the death of that person and/or others who may have died in similar circumstances. This means that there are very strict controls over cremations because exhumation is no longer possible and potential evidence is destroyed. Under the *Cremation (England and Wales) Regulations 2008*, the following forms must be completed:

- **Form 1:** This is the application for cremation, signed by a relative or executor.
- **Form 4 (medical certificate):** This is completed by the attending doctor who must have seen the body after death and he is paid a fee. He must attest whether any hazardous implants have been removed, e.g. pacemakers and if the death was referred to the coroner.
- **Form 5 (confirmatory medical certificate):** This is completed by a doctor of 5 or more years full registration, who must see the body after death and question the doctor who signed Form 4. He must not have been involved in the care of or be related to the deceased and he must have no known pecuniary interest. He must not be in partnership with or related to the other doctor and he also receives a fee. Note that the requirement for this form was suspended during the COVID-19 pandemic. This form is not necessary if the deceased died in hospital and a post mortem was performed.
- **Form 6:** This is issued by the coroner and replaces forms 4 and 5. It can be issued with or without an inquest but the cremation of people who died abroad requires authority from the Secretary of State. The Scottish equivalent is the Form E1.
- **Form 10:** This is the authority to cremate a body from the medical referee of the crematorium.
- **Form 11**: This is issued after a post mortem requested by the medical referee of the crematorium.

In Scotland, the statutory cremation forms are made under the *Cremation (Scotland) Regulations 2019* and cremations can only take place once the crematorium superintendent has received Form 14, which acknowledges that the death has been registered.

SUMMARY

This chapter covers both the practicalities and legalities of death. It lists who can confirm life extinct and explains how to do it properly. It takes the reader through accurate completion of the Medical Certificate of Cause of Death and the importance behind it. It then describes the new Medical Examiner system, which was brought in following the case of Harold Shipman and takes the reader through the different coronial systems of the United Kingdom—the Coroner in England, Wales and Northern Ireland and the Procurator Fiscal in Scotland It ends by discussing the various disposals for dead bodies and post mortems.

NOTES

1. Lewis, A., Cahn-Fuller, K., Caplan, A. Shouldn't dead be dead?: the search for a uniform definition of death. *J Law Med Ethics*. 2021;45(1):112–128.
2. See www.bma.org.uk/media/2323/bma-guidelines-for-remote-voed-april-2020.pdf.
3. Rutty, G.N., Duerden. R.M., Carter. N., Clark. J.C. Are Coroners' necropsies necessary? A prospective study examining whether a 'view & grant' system of death certification could be introduced into England & Wales. *J Clin Pathol*. 2001;54(4):279–284.
4. *The Shipman inquiry Third report, Death Certification and the Investigation of Deaths by Coroners*: Cm 5854 July 2003.
5. See www.england.nhs.uk/establishing-medical-examiner-system-nhs/.

FURTHER READING

Confirmation & Certification of Death. Guidelines for General Practitioners in England and Wales. General Practitioner Committee. British Medical Association, 2009.
Saukko, P., Knight. B. *Knight's forensic pathology*. 4th edn. CRC Press; 2015.

USEFUL WEBSITES

The Coroner system: www.cps.gov.uk/legal-guidance/coroners
The Procurator Fiscal system: https://www.copfs.gov.uk/

CHAPTER 12

Brain Stem Death and Organ Donation

INTRODUCTION

If the brain stem is irreversibly damaged, the centres that control breathing and circulation fail and the patient dies. This is known as 'brain stem death' (BSD) and is the point at which mechanical life support should be discontinued and retrieval of organs for transplantation considered. This chapter describes the criteria that must be satisfied in order to make a diagnosis of BSD and the tests performed. It further discusses the issues surrounding organ retrieval and transplantation.

DEFINITION OF DEATH

There is no statutory definition of death in the United Kingdom, but it can be regarded as 'irreversible loss of the capacity for consciousness, combined with irreversible loss of the capacity to breathe'.[1] This is the clinical state that follows BSD, so BSD equates with the death of the patient.

MAKING THE DIAGNOSIS OF BSD
Identification and Cause of Coma

BSD should only be considered where there is no doubt that the patient's condition is due to irremediable brain damage of known aetiology and it must not be confused with the problems relating to the diagnosis and management of permanent vegetative state (PVS) (see Chapter 13). BSD may be diagnosed

within hours, e.g. following a severe head injury, but it may take much longer, e.g. a patient who has suffered an indefinite period of cerebral hypoxia following a cardiac arrest. Other investigations such as a CT scan may be necessary to confirm the aetiology.

Exclusion of Other Causes of Coma
- **Hypothermia**—this can occur as a consequence, but it may also be the primary cause of loss of consciousness, so it is recommended that the core body temperature should be at least 34°C when the BSD tests are done.
- **Drugs**—those commonly used in the intensive therapy unit (ITU), such as benzodiazepines or opiates, can be cumulative and have prolonged action, particularly where the patient is hypothermic or is in renal or hepatic failure. These drugs must be stopped prior to the diagnosis being made. If the patient has no spontaneous respiration but received neuromuscular blocking agents, the persisting effects of these drugs must be excluded either by attempting to elicit the deep tendon reflexes or by demonstrating adequate neuromuscular conduction using a nerve stimulator.
- **Circulatory, metabolic and electrolyte imbalances**—some disturbances such as arrhythmias, diabetes insipidus and hypernatraemia may be a consequence of BSD but all potentially reversible disturbances should be excluded as the cause of the coma prior to making the diagnosis (Fig. 12.1).

BSD TESTS
BSD tests should be performed:
1. By two or more doctors who:
   - have been registered for 5 or more years
   - are competent in the field
   - are not members of the transplant team
   - at least one is a Consultant.
2. On two occasions by the two doctors—either separately or together—to reduce the risk of observer error and to confirm the irreversibility of the loss of the reflexes. There is no recommended set time period between the two sets of tests as it depends on the primary pathology and the state of the patient, but it should be adequate to reassure those

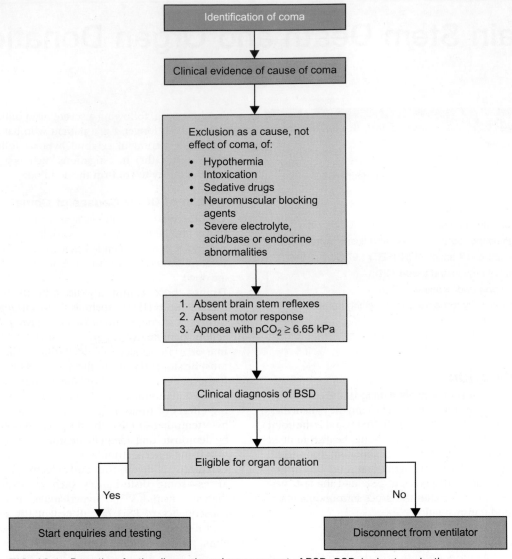

FIG. 12.1   Procedure for the diagnosis and management of BSD. *BSD*, brain stem death.

concerned. A minimum of 2 hours has been suggested, although in France there must be 24 hours between the two sets of tests. Please note Box 12.1 for the definitions of time of death.

3. On the first occasion that the patient has been observed to have fixed pupils and a complete absence of cranial nerve reflex responses for at least 4 hours.

The clinical criteria for BSD were established by the Conference of Colleges between 1976 and 1981[2] and they are:

1. **Absent brain stem reflexes**—note that it may be impossible to test all the reflexes in the presence of severe head and facial injuries. The tests shown in Table 12.1 are used to establish loss of the corresponding brain stem reflex.

TABLE 12.1
Tests to Establish Brain Stem Reflexes

Reflex	Test	Reflex Absent
Pupillary	Shine a *bright* light into each eye separately and observe for at least 1 minute	Pupils are fixed and do not constrict to light
Corneal	Lightly touch the cornea with cotton wool, taking care not to damage it	Eye does not blink
Vestibuloocular (Caloric)	Slowly inject ≥ 50 mL ice cold water over 1 minute into each external auditory meatus in turn with head flexed at 30 degrees. Check that auditory canals are clear prior to starting	Eyes do not move towards irrigated ear
Oculocephalic (Doll's eye)	Turn head rapidly from one side to the other while holding the eyes open and observe eye movement (omit if there is any risk of cervical spine damage)	Eyes move with the head and do not move within the orbit
Gag	Place suction catheter down trachea	No gagging or coughing

2. **Absent motor response**—no motor responses within the cranial nerve distribution can be elicited by adequate stimulation of any somatic area and there is no limb response to supraorbital pressure. Note that facial grimacing and spinal reflex movements of the limbs and torso may occur after BSD has been established and this may need to be explained to the relatives.

3. **Apnoea with pCO_2 ≥6.65 kPa**—the patient does not try to breathe once the ventilator has been disconnected and the threshold arterial pCO_2 for respiratory stimulation of 6.65 kPa has been reached. The preferred method is to ventilate the patient with 100% O_2 for 10 minutes, then with 5% CO_2 for 5 minutes. The ventilator should then be disconnected for 10 minutes and O_2 given at 8 L/min through a tracheal catheter to avoid hypoxia. The pCO_2 should be checked by measurement of the arterial blood gases but note that patients with preexisting respiratory disease may need much higher levels of pCO_2 before they are stimulated to breathe. Peripheral neurological syndromes must be excluded as a cause of the apnoea. This test should only be done after the other tests have confirmed BSD as the rise in pCO_2 provokes a rise in intracranial pressure that could endanger patients not yet dead.

The heart has been shown to stop beating a short period after fulfilment of these criteria, even if ventilation is continued.

Note that the criteria do not include results of tests such as CT scans or electroencephalograms (EEGs) as there is no evidence at present that they assist in the determination of brain stem death (BSD).

These criteria also apply in children of 2 months or older. It is only rarely possible to establish BSD in babies between 37 weeks gestation and 2 months. The criteria do not apply to babies that were born after less than 37 weeks' gestation. A Working Party of the Conference of Colleges on Organ Transplantation in Neonates recommended that organs could be removed from anencephalic infants when two doctors agree that spontaneous respiration has ceased.[3]

MANAGEMENT OF BSD

It is essential that the relatives are kept updated on the patient's condition and prognosis at all stages and that the tests are explained. All attempts to maintain adequate fluid intake, electrolyte balance and normal blood pressure should be continued until after BSD has been diagnosed and may be continued beyond that if the patient is to be an organ donor. Note that nontherapeutic (elective) ventilation is illegal as the patient does not benefit from it and it cannot be said to be in the patient's best interests, so it cannot be justified.

DONATION AFTER CARDIORESPIRATORY ARREST (DCD)

DCD is defined as retrieval of organs for transplantation from patients whose death has been diagnosed by cardiorespiratory criteria and there are two types:

1. **Controlled**—this occurs following the planned withdrawal of life-sustaining treatment (see Chapter 13).
2. **Uncontrolled**—this follows a sudden cardiac arrest from which the patient either cannot or should not be resuscitated.

DCD has increased in the last decade in the United Kingdom, mainly due to the increase in controlled DCD and now accounts for 40% of all deceased organ donors. The ischaemic injury means that fewer organs can be harvested but DCD is an important source of kidneys. In the United Kingdom, there are currently no programmes for organ retrieval following uncontrolled cardiorespiratory arrest.

MANAGEMENT OF POTENTIAL ORGAN AND TISSUE DONORS

In order for a patient to become an organ donor, they must fulfil the following criteria:

1. BSD or in established cardiorespiratory arrest and maintained on a ventilator
2. No history of or risks for infection with HIV or hepatitis
3. No history of malignant disease except some primary brain tumours (although such patients may still donate tissue, e.g. cornea)
4. No undiagnosed systemic infection.

Identification of Potential Donors

Since this book was first written, the law has changed and now all patients are considered to be organ donors if they:

- Are over 18
- Have not 'opted out' by recording their decision on the Organ Donor Register that they do not wish to donate their organs
- Are not in an excluded group:
  - Those who lack the mental capacity to understand the system and their opportunity to opt out
  - UK visitors or those not living in the United Kingdom voluntarily
  - People who have been resident in the United Kingdom less than 1 year.

In 2015, the *Human Transplantation (Wales) Act 2013* enabled an opt-out organ donation register in Wales, and England followed in 2020 after the enactment of the *Organ Donation (Deemed Consent) Act 2019*. Scotland joined in 2021 with the *Human Tissue (Authorisation) (Scotland) Act 2019* and the 'opt out' system will apply in Northern Ireland from 2023. The reason for the change is that the demand for organs has always outstripped the supply and advances in medical science have only made the gap bigger. Organ donation depends on the donor giving voluntary consent (see Chapter 5) and that can be to either 'opt in', e.g. carry a donor card or to not 'opt out', i.e. do not register as unwilling to donate their organs (deemed consent). Opt-out legislation can dramatically increase the number of organs available—Germany, which has the opt-in legislation has an organ donation consent rate of 12% whereas in Austria, which has opt-out laws it is 98.98%.[4] Deemed consent does not apply to children under 18 years and organ donation can only proceed with the consent of those with parental responsibility.

When a potential donor joins the Organ Donor Register, he can agree that any organ or tissue can be used or specify any or all of the following organs:

- heart
- lungs
- liver
- pancreas
- kidneys
- small bowel
- corneas.

These organs are listed as they are regarded as 'routine' transplants, which are the only transplants included under the opt-out system. Nonroutine transplants such as hands or face require specific opt-in consent from the family.

Donor Cards

Even if a patient carries a donor card or has made his wishes known by inclusion on the NHS Organ Donor Register, the family must still be consulted prior to harvesting the organs. Although they have no legal right to object, the NHS staff will respect their wishes if they do and the organs will not be taken, so it is important for all potential donors to discuss their decision with their family beforehand. Note that although the donor can specify which organs may be taken, neither he nor the relatives can impose any conditions on the use of the donated organs. An example of a current donor card is shown in Fig. 12.2.

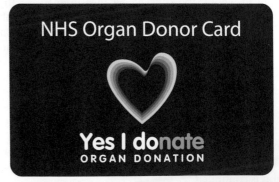

FIG. 12.2 Donor card. With permission from NHS Blood and Transplant. The NHS Organ Donor Card. Available at https://www.organdonation.nhs.uk/helping-you-to-decide/about-organ-donation/the-nhs-organ-donor-card/. Accessed 19 June 2023.

Specialist Nurse-Organ Donation (SN-OD)

The role of the SN-OD is to clinically assess the potential donor and inform and support the donor family, so he should ideally be involved from the initial end-of-life care decision (see Chapter 13). Once authorisation has been given, the SN-OD will coordinate the organ offering, retrieval and donor and donor family aftercare.

Recipient Transplant Coordinator (RTC)

The role of the RTC is to guide and support the recipient from the time of their first referral for consideration for a transplant to their aftercare post-transplant.

NHS BLOOD AND TRANSPLANT (NHSBT)

NHSBT is a special health authority, which was formed in 2005 by combining the National Blood (Transfusion) Service and UK Transplant. Its remit is to improve the supply and quality of donated organs, blood and other tissues to the NHS, so it has the following roles:

1. Encouraging people to donate and educating them in the process
2. Matching, allocating and distributing organs for transplant in a fair and transparent manner
3. Collecting, preparing and distributing of whole blood, plasma, platelet and cord blood donations
4. Supporting stem cell transplants and maintaining the Bone Marrow Registry
5. Operating the largest tissue bank in the United Kingdom and organising collection both pre, e.g. bone following a hip replacement, and post mortem, e.g. corneas
6. Providing diagnostic and therapeutic services
7. Maintaining the NHS Organ Donor Register, which contains the details of people willing to donate some or all their organs. In 2018, there were 25 million people on the register, which was 38% of the population
8. Running clinical trials and supporting research and development
9. Supporting transplant centres
10. Liaising with the SN-OD and RTC.

RETRIEVAL OF ORGANS AND TISSUE

In the United Kingdom, BSD donors will donate an average of 3.3 organs and DCD donors 2.7. The organ quality falls rapidly in donors over 50 years, especially hearts and lungs, but if the physiological status of the donor is optimised prior to retrieval, the number of suitable organs increases. Once death has been confirmed and authorisation given for organ removal, the SN-OD will contact the NHSBT and a National Organ Retrieval Services (NORS) team will be dispatched. The SN-OD will also organise the practical issues such as theatre time and any relevant screening tests. Malignant disease must also be excluded where possible although this is less important for certain types of tissue, e.g. corneal. Organ retrieval can start before the virology and bacteriology results are available, but the organs cannot be transplanted until they are pronounced clear of infection. The tissues that can be retrieved and stored for long periods following circulatory arrest are shown in Table 12.2.

ORGAN SUPPLY AND DEMAND

Organ transplantation is still the cheapest and most effective solution for end-stage organ failure but demand for organs continues to outstrip supply. In 2018 in the United Kingdom alone, 6000 patients were waiting for a transplant with three dying every day. The limited supply of organs has led to:

1. **Rationing**

   Rationing is inevitable but presents a serious ethical problem, as it is difficult to decide what parameters should be used and where the limit should lie, e.g. an age limit is likely to be very arbitrary and while a physically fit patient is more likely to survive the operation, it may provide a sicker patient with their only chance of survival. Questions have also been raised about the impact of lifestyle choices—should someone whose liver was destroyed by alcohol abuse be given the same priority as someone who needs a liver transplant for congenital reasons?

2. **Measures to increase the number of organs available**

   The following options have been considered or implemented but each presents their own unique ethical dilemmas:

   - **Opt-out system of organ donation**—see earlier.
   - **Living donors**—this is now accepted practice for some types of transplant, e.g. bone marrow and

TABLE 12.2 Tissue Storage Time Limits	
Tissue	**Time Limit (hours)**
Cornea	24
Skin	48
Bone	48
Heart valves	72

in the United Kingdom, more than 1000 people each year donate a kidney or part of their liver to both relatives and strangers. About 33% of kidney transplants are donated by living donors and they give the recipient a better outcome—the 10-year patient survival is 90% with a living donor transplant compared with 75% after one from a deceased donor. It also allows better planning of the operation and prior optimisation of the health of both the donor and the recipient. Donors must be in good health and certain conditions may preclude donation such as cancer, obesity, diabetes and hypertension. Most donors are related to the recipient but if they are not HLA-compatible, both donor and recipient can be entered into the paired or pooled donation scheme, which is run by the NHSBT. They can then be matched with one or more other pairs who are HLA-compatible. Altruistic donors, who are prepared to donate anonymously to a stranger, are entered into either the national transplant list or the Living Kidney Sharing Scheme. When a match is confirmed, the *Human Tissue Authority* must give permission for the transplant to go ahead and each pair must be assessed by an Independent Assessor to ensure that all the legal requirements are met. The NHSBT also ensures that there is no financial inducement or coercion being applied to the donor.

- **Xenotransplantation**—this is defined as the transfer of viable cells, tissues or organs between species. Some tissues, e.g. porcine heart valves and bovine insulin are already in common use, but the transplantation of whole organs is still in the early stages. The animal of choice is the pig, which breeds quickly with large litters, has organs of equivalent size and can be both genetically modified and reared in a pathogen-free environment. However, there are numerous technical difficulties and the risk of infection with foreign pathogens in a patient who has been immunocompromised to prevent graft rejection cannot be ignored. There is also the obvious dilemma as to whether it is morally acceptable to sacrifice an animal to save a human. Xenotransplantation in the United Kingdom was regulated by the UK Xenotransplantation Interim Regulatory Authority (UKXIRA), but it was disbanded in 2005.
- **Fetal tissue**—experimental work has already been done on the use of fetal pancreas as a treatment for diabetes and neural cells for Parkinson's disease with varying degrees of success. The procedures raise several ethical issues, including the source of the fetal tissue—whether from spontaneous or induced abortions—and whether or not the mother should be told of the intended use.
- **Payment for organs**—it is a criminal offence under the *Human Tissue Act 2004* (*2006* in Scotland) to make or receive a payment in return for supplying an organ for transplantation from a dead or living person. It is also an offence to arrange such a payment or advertise for donors with the promise of remuneration but 'organ trafficking' and 'transplant tourism' to poorer countries with no such legal protection still happens. Note that the term 'payment' does not include the costs of removing, transporting or preserving an organ, nor loss of earnings or reasonable expenses paid to a living donor.

DONATING A BODY TO BE USED FOR TEACHING PURPOSES

The deceased will normally have made advance arrangements to donate his body, so a written statement should be amongst his papers. Factors to be considered by the medical school prior to accepting the body include place and cause of death, the condition of the body, pre-existing illnesses and the demand for bodies. Bodies are usually refused if there has been a post mortem or if organs other than the corneas have been removed. They may be kept for teaching purposes for up to 3 years and then they are cremated or buried at a special memorial service with the costs borne by the medical school.

SUMMARY

This chapter covers the difficult and often controversial subjects of death and organ transplantation. It defines brain stem death (BSD) and sets out the tests required to establish BSD. It also discusses death following cardiorespiratory arrest and subsequent donation. It outlines the donation procedure and the current UK legislation regulating organ donation. It also describes the different options that have been considered to address the fact that organ demand outstrips supply and the process that follows donation of a whole body for medical teaching purposes.

NOTES

1. *A Code of Practice for the Diagnosis of Brain Stem Death.* Department of Health, 2008.
2. Criteria for the diagnosis of brain stem death. *J R Col Phys* 1995;21:381–382.
3. Working party on organ transplantation in neonates: Conference of Medical Colleges and Faculties of the United Kingdom. London DHSS, 1988.
4. Johnson, E.J., Goldstein, D.G. Do defaults save lives? *Science.* 2003;302(5649):1338–1339.

FURTHER READING

A Code of Practice for the Diagnosis and Confirmation of Death. Academy of Medical Royal Colleges, 2008.

USEFUL WEBSITES

Organ Donation and Transplantation: www.odt.nhs.uk
NHS Blood and Transplant: www.nhsbt.nhs.uk
Human Tissue Authority: www.hta.gov.uk

CHAPTER 13

Euthanasia, Withdrawing Treatment and Advance Decisions

INTRODUCTION

There has been much confusion over the terms 'euthanasia' and 'withdrawing or withholding treatment', but the simplest distinction is that euthanasia involves an active intervention to end life whereas withdrawal of treatment means not attempting to prolong life. Most countries still believe that passive euthanasia, i.e. letting a patient die is acceptable whereas active euthanasia, i.e. killing is not, but there has been a shift from refusal of treatment to a request for aid to die. In the United Kingdom, healthcare professionals (HCPs) have a moral and legal obligation to act upon a valid Advance Decision (AD) that refuses treatment but if 'assisted dying' ever does become lawful, HCPs may find themselves at least having to consider that same obligation to assist a patient's death.

EUTHANASIA

Introduction

Euthanasia has been defined as 'procuring a painless and easy death', although the NHS website describes it as 'the act of deliberately ending a person's life to relieve suffering' and its legalisation has been the subject of much heated discussion. It has furious opposition but also fervent supporters and has stimulated many legal, ethical, moral and religious debates.

There are four forms of euthanasia:

1. **Voluntary active**—a competent adult asks a third party to help them to die. If the third party agrees, this is assisted suicide.
2. **Voluntary passive**—a competent adult dies following withdrawal of treatment at their request.
3. **Involuntary passive**—treatment is withdrawn or withheld from a patient who lacks capacity in their 'best interests' (see Chapter 5), e.g. unconscious or comatose.
4. **Involuntary active**—this is murder!

History

Existing laws allow terminally ill people to request the removal of life-sustaining medical interventions and to receive palliative drugs that may speed up death. In 1996, an Appeals Court in America held that those who wished to hasten their death but were not dependent on life-sustaining technology were unequally treated, so physician-assisted suicide should be made legally available. The following year, the Supreme Court of the United States ruled that 'the right to commit suicide with another's assistance' was not a constitutional right and not the same as the right to refuse treatment. However, it also said that physician-assisted suicide was not unconstitutional and that each State could decide the issue on an individual basis. The preferred term for **physician-assisted suicide** is now **physician-assisted dying** and it occurs when a doctor prescribes a lethal drug, but it is administered by the patient himself. Studies have shown that doctors prefer the concept of physician-assisted dying as it confers a more passive role and use of the term 'dying' is more socially acceptable than 'suicide'.

Legal Position in Other Countries

The countries where assisted suicide is either not unlawful or currently legal under specified and often varied circumstances are:

- Australia (Victoria)
- Belgium—*Belgian Euthanasia Act 2002*
- Canada (Quebec since 2014; nationwide as of June 2016)—*Medical Assistance in Dying Act 2016*
- Colombia
- Holland—*Termination of Life on Request and Assisted Suicide (Review Procedures) Act 2001*
- Luxembourg—*Law on the Right to Die with Dignity 2008*

- Switzerland—euthanasia is illegal but assisted suicide is lawful as long as there are no 'self-seeking motives'—Article 115 of the *Swiss Penal Code 1937*
- Parts of the USA:
  - California—*California End of Life Option Act 2015*
  - Colorado—*End of Life Options Act 2016*
  - Hawaii—*Hawaii Death with Dignity Act 2018*
  - Maine—*Maine Death with Dignity Act 2019*
  - New Jersey—*New Jersey Dignity in Dying Bill of Rights Act 2019*
  - Oregon—*Oregon Death with Dignity Act 1994*— the first law that allowed assisted dying
  - Vermont—*Patient Choice and Control at End of Life Act 2013*
  - Washington—*Washington Death with Dignity Act 2008*
  - Washington DC—*District of Columbia Death with Dignity Act 2016*
  - (It was also briefly legal in New Mexico in 2014, but it was overturned in 2015).

In most countries, people who want to die using the assisted suicide model will only qualify for it if they meet certain criteria including:

- Being an adult of 18 or over
- Having a terminal illness
- Being of sound mind
- Voluntarily and repeatedly expressing their wish to die
- Able to take the specified, lethal dose of drugs themselves.

Belgium has been declared as the country with the most relaxed approach to voluntary euthanasia after the *Belgian Euthanasia Act 2002* was extended in 2014 to include mental disabilities as well as physical ones, children without any age limit and criminals. This means that it is the only European country that allows children to be euthanised at any age, unlike Holland, where the minor must be older than 12 years and Luxembourg, where the child must be over 16 and, if under 18, must also obtain the authority of their parent or legal guardian. Outside Europe, only adults 18 years or older can request assisted suicide and only physician-assisted suicide is lawful, except in Colombia. In 2015, Colombia passed a resolution to allow euthanasia in adults, although the practice had been allowed since 1997 without any penalties. In March 2018, it became the third country to allow euthanasia of minors, although they must have a life-limiting condition to be eligible. If the child is aged 6 to 12, he must be evaluated by a psychiatrist to ensure that he understands his choice and his parents or legal guardian must also consent; if he is aged between 12 and 14,

he can request the procedure with parental consent and children over 14 can request an assisted death, even if their parents do not agree.

Legal Position in the United Kingdom

Following the introduction of the *Suicide Act* in 1961, it is no longer illegal to take one's own life, but it is still an offence to encourage or assist someone else to take their life, punishable by up to 14 years in prison, even if that person requests that assistance. This means that people who wish to choose the mode and time of their death must either enlist amateur help or travel to countries where physician-assisted dying is not illegal. In 2018, 43 people from the United Kingdom died at two facilities in Switzerland, Dignitas and Life Circle, and research by Dignity in Dying found that there was an average of 14,800 internet searches for 'Dignitas' every month in the United Kingdom.[1]

The case of Diane Pretty,[2] who was terminally ill from motor neurone disease (MND) first raised the question of legalisation of assisted dying for the terminally ill in the United Kingdom in 2002. She wanted her husband to be allowed to help her to die when she felt that her life was no longer tolerable and she needed a guarantee from the Director of Public Prosecutions (DPP) that he would not be prosecuted as a result. The case went all the way to the House of Lords and the European Court of Human Rights before ultimately deciding that she did not have a right to be assisted to die and Mrs Pretty died aged 43 from the consequences of her MND 2 weeks after the final judgement. There have been many common law cases and attempts to pass bills on assisted dying through Parliament since then, but assisted dying remains illegal in the United Kingdom, although the British Medical Association (BMA) have recently changed their stance and are no longer strictly opposed to it.

There remains a clear distinction between an active act to end life ('killing the patient') and a passive act, such as withdrawing or withholding treatment ('letting him die'), but an active act could still be acceptable if it encompasses the 'doctrine of double effect'. This is when a drug is given, which has palliative and/or therapeutic advantage but that may, in conjunction with other factors, result in the death of the patient. An example of this is morphine, which relieves the distressing shortness of breath in patients suffering from cardiac failure, as it reduces the work of the heart, but it has an associated side effect of respiratory depression, so it can either improve the patient's breathing or stop it depending on the circumstances, which may be difficult to predict. However, the doctrine of double effect relies on the distinction between intention and foresight, which is not recognised on UK law and clinicians cannot use it as a defence if it is found that the drug was given in nontherapeutic doses. If the drug given, e.g. potassium chloride or other action taken has no medical, palliative or therapeutic use and is intended purely to end life, then it is murder and cannot be justified.

It has been suggested that if euthanasia was legalised, then there would be greater safeguards while others fear that legalisation would allow uninhibited involuntary euthanasia. Data from Oregon and the Netherlands do not support either argument.

WITHDRAWAL OF TREATMENT
Permanent Vegetative State (PVS)
PVS is distinct from brain stem death (see Chapter 12) in that the brain stem still functions while the cortex does not. This means that the patient can breathe unaided and the autonomic nervous system works but he cannot see, hear, speak, feel pain or move voluntarily, although he still has reflex movement. It is diagnosed when the following criteria have been satisfied[3]:

1. The patient shows no evidence of awareness of self or his environment following repeated examinations by a specially trained assessor.
2. There is established brain damage of known cause, consistent with the diagnosis.
3. There are no reversible causes present, e.g. drugs or metabolic disorders.
4. There are no treatable causes, e.g. an operable brain tumour.
5. Over 6 months have passed since a nontraumatic brain injury, e.g. a stroke and over 12 months since a traumatic one.

However, the diagnosis of PVS cannot be absolutely certain, data on prognosis are limited and there is no standard test of awareness so there are many ethical issues surrounding the withdrawal of treatment.

Principles of Withdrawal of Treatment
- HCPs draw a distinction between withdrawing and withholding treatment, but most courts do not.
- If there is a possibility that the patient will receive benefit from the treatment, it should be continued and effective palliation should never be withdrawn.
- The decision to stop treatment must be on the basis that to continue would be futile, or not in the patient's best interests, not because the patient has

become incompetent and it should never be denied on the basis of cost.
- The autonomy of the patient must be respected and basic care and nutrition should continue, although tube feeding may be regarded as a treatment and can be stopped where there is no chance of recovery.
- If the patient has a valid AD (see later) declining treatment, it must be followed.
- If the patient has given someone legal power of attorney for healthcare matters (see Chapter 16), their instructions must be followed where clinically appropriate, although they cannot advocate treatment against medical advice.
- Communication with the relatives is vital and although the doctors should make the final decision, it is advisable to seek their agreement.
- If there is no legal proxy and no one who may know the patient's final wishes, the clinician in charge should request that the local authority appoint an Independent Mental Capacity Advocate (IMCA— see Chapter 16), as required by the *Mental Capacity Act 2005*.
- Guidance from the Court of Protection (see Chapter 16) may be sought before withholding life-prolonging treatment, but it is no longer essential.
- The reasons for deciding to withdraw treatment must be clearly, comprehensively, contemporaneously and accurately recorded in the notes.
- 20% of people admitted to critical care die and withdrawal of treatment accounts for 60% of those deaths.

Legal Position
The landmark case in the debate about withdrawal of treatment was that of *Airedale NHS Trust v Bland 1992/3*.[4] Anthony Bland was left in PVS after being crushed in the Hillsborough Football Stadium disaster of April 1989. The Trust and the family asked the court if it would be lawful to discontinue clinically assisted nutrition and hydration (CANH) and any further medical treatment, as the situation was hopeless and it would lead to his death. The court agreed but the Official Solicitor appealed on behalf of Anthony and it was upheld in the Court of Appeal. The Trust and family appealed to House of Lords where it was decided that the principle of sanctity of life is not absolute and does not compel a doctor to feed a patient against his will or keep a terminally ill patient alive against their wishes. There is just as much duty to discontinue as to continue treatment and the decision must be based on what the patient would have wished had he been able to decide. The court ruled that CANH was

a treatment and that a decision to withhold a life-sustaining treatment would not *necessarily* lead to criminal liability.

Since 2018, HCPs no longer have to apply to the Court of Protection for permission to withdraw CANH from patients in a PVS, as long as the family and clinical staff agree and it is in the best interests of the patient.

ADVANCE STATEMENTS AND DECISIONS
Introduction
An Advance Statement is a statement made by a mentally competent adult that gives instructions about how he would wish to be treated in the event of any future loss of capacity. An Advance Decision (AD) is a decision made by a mentally competent adult to refuse a specific type of treatment in the future and it is also known as a 'Living Will' or an advance decision to refuse treatment (ADRT). Both Advance Statements and Decisions may be seen as a method of extending a person's autonomy by allowing them to make or convey decisions from which they would otherwise have been excluded on the basis of their incapacity. Competence, capacity and methods of assessment are discussed in Chapter 5.

Legal Position
ADs were first introduced in America in 1967. American healthcare is predominantly private and resource driven, so doctors tend to be far more interventional than those in the United Kingdom. ADs were proposed as a method of restricting the number of invasive procedures being imposed on patients who did not want them. The Voluntary Euthanasia Society (now called Dignity in Dying) followed suit in the United Kingdom in the early 1970s but with a greater emphasis on patient choice. Initially, the close association of ADs with the euthanasia movements limited their use but they became more widely accepted once they were seen as a method of exercising autonomy rather than simply the right to die. The first statutory support came in the *Natural Death Act of California* in 1976 and now most American States have a statutory obligation to allow ADs. There is also federal legislation in the form of the *Patient Self-Determination Act 1991*, which compels hospitals and nursing homes to give patients the opportunity to make an AD at the time of admission.

It took far longer for ADs to become legally binding in the United Kingdom. In 1993, a patient's advance refusal of treatment became legally binding under common law (see Chapter 2) with the ruling that a schizophrenic inpatient of Broadmoor could refuse amputation of his gangrenous leg then and at any time in the future, even if he became incompetent.[5] In the same year, in the case of Bland (see earlier), the judges stated that if he had made an AD prior to his injury, it would have been legally binding.

In 1995, the Law Commission endorsed 'advance statements about health' and recommended legislation, with statute law clearly stipulating how competent adults could control their future care. Later that year a code of practice for ADs was published jointly by the BMA and the Royal Colleges of Nursing, Physicians and General Practitioners.[6] In 1999, the NHS Executive issued guidance on withholding consent to treatment[7] and this was closely followed by guidance from the General Medical Council (GMC) on the legal position of ADs.[8]

ADs to refuse treatment are now legally binding in the United Kingdom if they are 'valid and applicable under the requirements of the *Mental Capacity Act 2005*' (see Chapter 16) and both the Act and its associated Code of Practice make it clear that the responsibility for an AD lies with the person making it. Advance statements are **not** legally binding but must be followed when making 'best interests' judgements.

An AD will have legal standing if the conditions set out in Box 13.1 are met.

Types
There are many different types of ADs, but they must be written and cannot be verbal if refusing life-sustaining

---

BOX 13.1
Conditions

1. The author had capacity, was over 18 and was not under any duress at the time of completion.
2. The author was fully informed about the nature and possible consequences of an AD at the time of completion, especially the risk to life.
3. The situations to which the AD applies are clearly stated and now apply.
4. Responsibility for that decision has not been subsequently conferred onto a lasting power of attorney for healthcare matters.
5. The AD has not been amended or revoked.
6. The author now lacks the capacity to make his own decision.
7. The AD refuses certain treatments or specifies the level of deterioration at which active treatment should cease.
8. It is signed and witnessed.

treatment. Compassion in Dying provides an AD template in pdf format that can be completed online or downloaded from its website, along with instructions on its use.

The Scope and Limitations of Advance Decisions

Under the *Mental Capacity Act 2005* Code of Practice, HCPs will be protected from liability if:

- They stop or withhold treatment because they reasonably believe that a valid and applicable AD exists.
- Start or continue treatment if they do not know that an AD exists or do not believe it to be valid and applicable, but they cannot deliberately ignore a valid AD or they risk prosecution.
- If they have started treatment in the emergency situation but stop once presented with a valid and applicable AD.
- A valid AD:
  - To refuse treatment has the same legal status as a patient with capacity to refuse treatment and deserves the same respect.
  - Cannot dictate the type or amount of treatment that a patient should receive. The patients' wishes should be considered but treatment remains a clinical decision.
  - Should not preclude the provision of basic care, defined as the maintenance of bodily cleanliness, relief of sustained and serious pain, and the provision of oral nutrition and hydration, although it can be used to refuse CANH, as this is legally a treatment.

If the HCP has a reasonable belief that the AD is not valid, he must still consider the wishes expressed in the AD when making a 'best interests' decision and if he does not feel able to comply with a valid AD, he has an obligation to transfer the care of that patient to another HCP. If there is a disagreement between HCPs or between the HCP and the family about the validity of an AD, it may require recourse to the Court of Protection to resolve the dispute.

Note that a patient cannot refuse treatment:

- That has been required by law
- If his condition would put others at risk.

There are some special circumstances:

- People under 18 years cannot make ADs, but the *Children Act 1989* emphasises that their wishes must be considered when deciding on their treatment if they have reached the level of 'Gillick competence' (see Chapter 5).

- A patient detained under the *Mental Health Act 1983* can make a valid AD providing that he has capacity to do so, but only about those treatments not specified under the terms of their detention.
- If a woman is pregnant when her AD becomes valid, then the needs of the fetus supersede compliance with it, but the case should still be referred to the Court of Protection.

Note that an AD cannot be used to:

- Request treatment, although the patient can express their wishes for their future care in their Advance Statement, but this is not legally binding.
- Authorise treatment that is illegal, e.g. assisting the patient to commit suicide.

Advantages of Advance Decisions

1. They recognise the autonomy of the patient and give him peace of mind.
2. The HCPs are reassured that they are providing the type of care that the patient would have wanted without fear of possible future legal redress.
3. They provide an opportunity for HCPs to discuss future management with the patient and the relatives as part of the advance care planning process.
4. They relieve the relatives of making decisions for which they do not wish to be responsible.
5. They can be amended or revoked in whole or in part at any time while the patient still has capacity and made more applicable to the patients' condition and likely future interventions.

Disadvantages of Advance Decisions

1. Assessment of capacity may be difficult and subject to later criticism.
2. Refusal of treatment must be fully informed, but it can only be valid if the facts relating to the current situation are available.
3. Advances in medical treatment may invalidate an AD by changing the situations to which it applies.
4. Refusal of a particular intervention may have consequences other than death, e.g. an asthmatic who refuses ventilation may not die but could suffer hypoxic brain damage.
5. ADs only cover refusal of treatment and other factors may be equally important to the patient such as place of death.
6. Conservatism—it is easier to do something than nothing, particularly in situations when failure to

> **BOX 13.2**
> **Criteria for the Patient**
>
> 1. Has capacity—this must be presumed unless there is evidence to the contrary
> 2. Is aware of the legal standing
> 3. Is able to understand the implications
> 4. Can accurately foresee possible future circumstances in which it might apply
> 5. Is fully informed about his diagnosis, prognosis and possible treatments
> 6. Is aware of potential future advances in the treatment of his disease
> 7. Is aware that the AD can be amended or revoked at any time
> 8. Has plans to regularly review the AD
> 9. Is not under any duress.

treat cannot be reversed and may result in litigation or other unforeseen consequences.

Making an Advance Decision

If you are asked to witness or help compose an AD, you should ensure that the criteria set out in Box 13.2 have been met.

Patients should be discouraged from making ADs when they are acutely unwell or soon after being given a poor prognosis. They should also be told that it is their responsibility to ensure that any HCP involved in their future care is made aware of the existence of the AD. If the AD refuses any form of life-sustaining treatment, it must be signed and witnessed.

Warning! If the AD appears to be valid, comply with the refusal of treatment. If there is ANY doubt, act in the 'best interests' of the patient and seek further advice.

Cardiopulmonary Resuscitation (CPR) and Do Not Attempt CPR (DNACPR)

If the healthcare team decides that there is no realistic prospect of CPR having a successful outcome, they will either not offer or not attempt it. This is a clinical decision and does not require an AD to authorise it. Patients can also decide in advance that they do not want CPR and request that a DNACPR order is placed in their medical notes.

SUMMARY

This chapter covers the emotive subjects of euthanasia, assisted suicide or dying, withdrawing or withholding treatment, persistent vegetative state and advance decisions and statements. It defines each subject before outlining the history, progress and current legal position in both the United Kingdom and worldwide. It presents a balanced view of often very controversial topics and also clarifies the situation with regard to the 'doctrine of double effect'. It then educates the reader on the best ways to assess and manage a patient who has made an Advance Decision and how to ensure that the Advance Decision is 'valid and applicable under the requirements of the *Mental Capacity Act 2005*'.

CASE SCENARIOS

1. You are on duty in the emergency department and a 65-year-old man is brought in with severe difficulty in breathing as a result of his end-stage motor neurone disease (MND). He is accompanied by his wife, who hands you an Advance Decision (AD), which she says he made 5 years ago. In it, your patient apparently declines 'life-sustaining treatment' but does not specify what. She says that she will support any decision made by the healthcare staff, but she does not want to be involved, as she would rather he was treated but respects his wishes. You note that the AD is not signed or witnessed so should you and/or can you start treatment?

2. You speak to his wife who tells you that he wrote the AD after watching his sister die a protracted death on intensive therapy unit (ITU) after a respiratory arrest and he was adamant that he did not want to be put on a ventilator. She still does not want to be involved and would like you to wait for the arrival of their son if possible, who is his father's lasting power of attorney (LPA) for health matters. Should you stop treatment?

3. The patient's son arrives with the LPA authorisation and a new copy of the AD, which has been signed, witnessed and dated within the past month. In this AD, the patient clearly states that he does not want to be ventilated 'under any circumstances' and that he is aware that this might result in his death. The son would like you to stop treatment—should you?

See 'Answers to case scenarios'.

NOTES

1. BBC News. What's the difference between assisted suicide and euthanasia? 8 February 2019.
2. *R (Pretty) v Director of Public Prosecutions* [2002] 1 AC 800 [2001] UKHL 61.

3. Wade, D.T. Ethical issues in diagnosis and management of patients in the permanent vegetative state. *BMJ.* 2001;322:352–354.
4. *Airedale NHS Trust v Bland* [1993] 1 All ER 821, (1993) 12 BMLR 64.
5. *Re C* [1994] 1 All ER 819, (1993) 15 BMLR 77.
6. British Medical Association. *Advance statements about medical treatment. Code of practice and explanatory notes.* London: BMA; 1995.
7. NHS Executive. *Consent to treatment; summary of legal rulings.* London: NHSE; 1999 (Health Service Circular 1999/031).
8. General Medical Council. *Seeking patient's consent: the ethical considerations.* London: GMC; 1999.

FURTHER READING

General Medical Council. Treatment and care towards the end of life: good practice in decision making. Available at www. gmc-uk.org/-/media/documents/treatment-and-care-towards-the-end-of-life---english-1015_pdf-48902105.pdf.

The National Council for Palliative Care. Advance decisions to refuse treatment—a guide for health and social care professionals. Available at https://www.bl.uk/collection-items/advance-decisions-to-refuse-treatment-a-guide-for-health-and-social-care-professionals.

USEFUL WEBSITES

Compassion in Dying: www.compassionindying.org.uk
Dignity in Dying: www.dignityindying.org.uk
Right To Life: www.righttolife.org.uk

Child Abuse and the Children Acts

INTRODUCTION

Child abuse is one of the most distressing areas in which a healthcare professional (HCP) may become involved. This chapter outlines those features in the history and examination of a child that should make the HCP suspicious that the injuries seen may not be accidental in origin. It also covers the laws that relate to children with a detailed discussion of the *Children Acts*. Child sexual abuse is covered in more detail in Chapter 15.

LEGAL ASPECTS

There are some laws that relate specifically to children.

Infanticide

This is the deliberate killing of an infant <12 months old, although deaths usually occur within hours or minutes of birth. The infant must have had a separate existence and death must have occurred as a result of an act of either deliberate commission or omission, but this may be very difficult to prove, especially if the birth was initially concealed. The *Infanticide Act 1938* allows courts in England and Wales to take a lenient view of a mother who kills her infant while the 'balance of her mind was disturbed by reason of her not having fully recovered from the effects of giving birth to the child, or by reason of the effect of lactation consequent upon the birth of the child'. The same applies in Northern Ireland under the *Infanticide Act (Northern Ireland) 1939*, but it is still regarded as child murder in Scotland.

Stillbirth

This is defined in the *Still-Birth (Definition) Act 1992* and the *Still-Births (Scotland) Act 1938* as an infant who was born after 24 weeks' gestation and never showed signs of life after being expelled from the mother. It affects 1:50 births and requires special certification to allow the collection of statistical data on the cause of death (Stillbirths Certificate—see Chapter 11). Note that fetuses born at less than 24 weeks are not registered.

Child Destruction

This is the killing of a fetus in utero after 28 weeks (*Infant Life Preservation Act 1929*).

Concealment of Birth

This is defined in s 60 of the *Offences against the Person Act 1861 (England & Wales)* and the *Concealment of Birth (Scotland) Act 1809* as the hiding of a body to conceal the fact of birth. The cause of death, viability and whether stillborn or alive are all immaterial.

Other offences apply for all ages:
- **Common assault**—this is threatening behaviour and carries a maximum penalty of 6 months' imprisonment or a fine.
- **Battery**—this is the infliction of personal violence (as for common assault).
- **Actual bodily harm (ABH)**—this is intentional assault occasioning physical injury, e.g. bruising (5 years).
- **Grievous bodily harm (GBH)**—this is intentional wounding resulting in a breach in the skin or GBH, e.g. a fracture (life, although this is rarely imposed).
- **Manslaughter** (life).
- **Murder** (life).
- **Sexual offences** (see Chapter 15).

TYPES OF CHILD ABUSE

Child abuse is the intentional harm or mistreatment of a child under 18 years of age and there are many different forms, which can occur in isolation or concurrently.

Physical Abuse

The child is deliberately injured or put at risk of harm. The diagnosis and typical injuries are discussed later but there are often also long-term mental and physical sequelae such as anxiety and depression, self-harm, drug and alcohol abuse, behavioural problems, including criminal activity and eating disorders.

Sexual Abuse

This is defined as exposing a child to any form of sexual activity and involves either contact with the child, e.g. fondling or penetration, or noncontact, e.g. exposure to pornography. It can occur in person or online. Another form of sexual abuse is exploitation, which includes the offences of grooming and trafficking. This is explored further in Chapter 15.

Emotional Abuse

This is the continuing emotional maltreatment of a child with the intention of deliberately frightening, humiliating, ignoring or isolating him. It is also known as psychological abuse and includes threatening, blaming, excluding, demeaning and manipulating behaviour. It is often difficult to diagnose but emotionally abused children classically lack confidence, struggle to keep friends and exhibit behavioural problems such as bed-wetting.

Neglect

Neglect is the ongoing failure to meet the basic needs of a child and there are four main types:

- **Physical**—this is failure to provide adequate food, fluids, shelter or supervision, so the child is unsafe.
- **Emotional**—the child does not receive the emotional support or stimulation they need.
- **Educational**—the child does not regularly attend school, if at all and is not home-schooled.
- **Medical**—the child does not receive adequate medical or dental care.

Neglect is very difficult to diagnose but neglected children are often hungry, underweight and have dirty, unseasonal clothes with poor hygiene. They may also have chronic health problems, bad teeth and scant language and social skills.

Munchausen Syndrome by Proxy

This is also called factitious disorder imposed on another (FDIA) and it is an uncommon form of abuse, but it carries a high morbidity and mortality with a high incidence of reabuse. The caregiver, usually the mother, either deliberately makes the child ill or fabricates the symptoms. The child is then subjected to a series of investigations, which often makes the situation worse and the eventual diagnosis even more difficult. The commonest presentations are fits, bleeding, diarrhoea, vomiting, fever and rashes.

Female Genital Mutilation

This is the deliberate cutting, alteration or removal of the female genitalia for no medical reason and it is usually performed on prepubertal girls for reasons of tradition. It is illegal in England, Wales and Northern Ireland under the *Female Genital Mutilation Act 2003* and in Scotland under the *Prohibition of Female Genital Mutilation (Scotland) Act 2005*.

Child Trafficking and Modern Slavery

Most children involved in the modern slave trade are brought into the United Kingdom from abroad, especially Vietnam, Africa, Albania and Romania, but it can also happen within the United Kingdom. Children are forced, tricked or bribed to leave home, then trafficked around the United Kingdom for:

- sexual exploitation
- forced labour in factories, shops and domestic homes
- benefit fraud
- criminal activities, e.g. drug dealing, begging, stealing and cannabis farms.

Trafficked children are at a very high risk of all forms of child abuse, which may be used as a way of controlling them. This is a vast subject beyond the scope of this book, but any reader wanting more information about the signs, risks and effects of this abhorrent trade is recommended to access the 'Every Child Protected Against Trafficking' (ECPAT) website provided at the end of this chapter.

DIAGNOSIS OF CHILD ABUSE

HCPs are often reluctant to make a diagnosis of child abuse for fear of 'getting it wrong' but the following points in the history and examination of any child should make the HCP suspicious of nonaccidental injury (NAI):

History

1. **History inconsistent with injury**—the story given must match the type of injury, e.g. a cigarette burn is not caused by a boiling cup of tea.

TABLE 14.1
Risk Factors for Child Abuse

Parents or Guardians	Child
Domestic abuse	Premature
Young/immature parents	'Wrong' sex
Abused in childhood themselves	Sick children
Denied request for termination of pregnancy	Any abnormality—especially learning difficulties and deafness
Sporadic or no antenatal attendance	Multiple births
No access to professional support	Under 2 years of age
Cohabitee is not the parent of the child	Both boys and girls
Unemployed or made redundant	First born
Further pregnancies	
Drug and/or alcohol abuse	
Illness, especially mental	
No social support	

2. **History inconsistent with developmental milestones**—a 6-week-old baby cannot 'roll off the bed'.
3. **Varying or changing explanations**—the child may give a different explanation if he is interviewed in the absence of the parents, as may each parent. The story may also change as the family sees different HCPs.
4. **Delay in reporting the injury**—old injuries should raise suspicions unless there is a reasonable explanation for the delay such as a holiday abroad or that the child has been with a different carer. This is particularly important when there are multiple injuries of different ages.
5. **'Hospital hopping'**—abusive parents often take their children to different agencies, including different GP surgeries in an effort to avoid the child being highlighted as a frequent attendee. They may also give different names and details (Table 14.1).

Examination

1. **Fear of one or both parents**—abused children may appear frightened, but conversely, they may be excessively affectionate towards the parent in an effort to gain approval.

2. **Poor eye contact**—this is commonly seen in people who are not telling the truth and may involve the child and/or the carer.
3. **'Frozen awareness'**—this is a classic trait in children who have been abused over a long period, denoting a child who is either incapable or fearful of displaying any emotion.
4. **Excessive compliance with examination**—children are naturally shy and usually reluctant to undress in front of strangers. Abused children are often overly eager to comply with any instructions given.
5. **Seeking comfort from staff**—any child who prefers to be comforted by staff rather than the carer must be examined carefully for signs of abuse.
6. **Multiple injuries of differing ages**—all children get injured accidentally and may have multiple injuries, but they are usually minor and always on exposed prominent areas such as knees and elbows. However, the carer or child should still be asked for explanations for any injuries seen and a note made of any previous attendances for the more serious injuries.
7. **Different types of injury**—this is particularly important if all the injuries are of a similar age.
8. **Multiple injuries from single cause**, e.g. cigarette burns.

TYPES OF INJURIES
Surface Injuries
Some surface injuries are diagnostic of child abuse, whereas others are suspicious but must be viewed in conjunction with other signs. These are classic injuries:
- **Black eyes**—children rarely get black eyes accidentally.
- **'Tin ear'**—this is bruising of the pinna caused by a slap to the side of the head.
- **Slap marks**—these are linear petechial marks, often in the shape of a hand and commonly seen on the face.
- **Torn frenulum in babies**—this is caused by a bottle being forced into the mouth, usually in an attempt to stop the baby from crying.
- **Bruising around mouth**—this is indicative of smothering and again it is usually done in an attempt to silence the child.
- **Subconjunctival haemorrhages**—these indicate smothering, attempted strangulation and/or shaking.
- **Bald patches**—from hair pulling.

Bruises
All children (and many adults) have bruises and they are often multiple, but the following should raise suspicions of a nonaccidental origin:

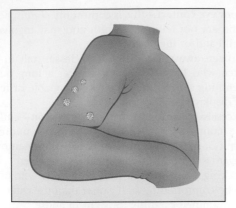

FIG. 14.1   Spot bruises on the upper arm.

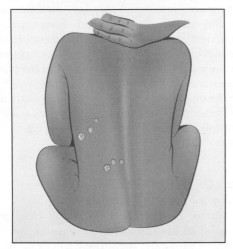

FIG. 14.2   Knuckle punches.

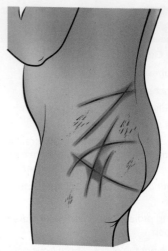

FIG. 14.3   Tramline bruising following beating with a stick.

- **Spot bruises**—these suggest pinch and fingertip marks. They are most commonly found on the limbs, chest and abdomen (Fig. 14.1).
- **Knuckle punches**—these are rows of three or four round bruises (Fig. 14.2).
- **Characteristic patterns**—some bruises have distinctive shapes that reflect the implement used, e.g. tramline bruising from sticks, belt buckle marks (Fig. 14.3).
- **Bruising in inaccessible areas**, e.g. inner thighs, spine or face in babies less than 18 months.

Bites

Bite marks are distinctive crescentic bruises, often found on the buttocks or limbs and usually multiple. It is important to distinguish adult bites from those of children—juvenile bites are smaller with a narrower arch. It is also essential to distinguish human bites from animal ones—humans make more use of the molars so there is more bruising and less piercing of the skin.

Burns

Children often burn themselves accidentally but 10% of abused children are burnt. Unless there is other pathology such as epilepsy, deep burns in children are almost exclusively due to abuse, as they signify prolonged contact with the offending object. Certain types of burns are characteristic of child abuse:

- **'Dipping' scalds**—these are scalds that are confined to the buttocks and heels, where the child has been dipped in boiling water. The usual story given is that the child sat down in a hot bath but if that were true, the child would also have scalds to the top of the feet and it is very unlikely that the child would then have sat down (Fig. 14.4).
- **Cigarette burns**—these are circular burns that are frequently full-thickness. They are usually multiple and often in exposed areas (Fig. 14.5).
- **Friction burns**—these indicate that the child has been dragged or tied up.
- **Burns in nonexposed areas or multiple burns from the same source**, e.g. from domestic iron.

Skeletal

Unlike accidental injuries, deliberate skeletal injuries usually occur as a result of torsion, angulation or traction rather than direct impact. Abused children often have multiple fractures of varying ages and they occur in sites that are rarely injured accidentally, e.g.

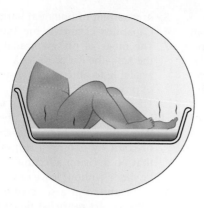

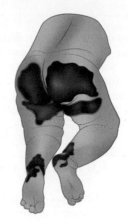

FIG. 14.4 Dipping scalds.

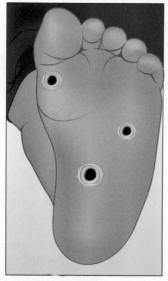

FIG. 14.5 Cigarette burns.

limbs in nonwalking babies and ribs. Rib fractures in a child under 5 years old are pathognomonic of abuse by squeezing and the chest X-ray may show the classic 'string of beads' appearance of the healing calluses. Metaphyseal chipping suggests shaking and areas of periosteal calcification denote 'near fractures', i.e. that a force has been applied but it was not sufficient to actually break the bone. Other skeletal injuries such as spiral diaphyseal and epiphyseal fractures can occur accidentally but are much more common in abused children.

Head Injuries

Head injuries are the commonest cause of death from abuse and over 95% of serious head injuries in children under 1 year old are nonaccidental. They range from bruises, abrasions and lacerations to more serious intracranial bleeds such as subdural haematomas and subarachnoid haemorrhages. Abused children also have a higher incidence of cerebral contusions, which are linked to learning difficulties and if there are associated retinal haemorrhages, this indicates a shaking component to the abuse (see later). Skull fractures occur most frequently in the occipito-parietal area whatever the cause, but an infant must fall at least 4 feet onto a hard surface to cause a skull fracture and diffuse brain injury.[1] This means that a story that the child with a skull fracture 'rolled off the bed' is unlikely to be true.

Shaken Baby Syndrome (SBS)

In 1946, Caffey first described shaken baby syndrome (SBS) as a clinical and pathological entity characterised by retinal and subdural and/or subarachnoid haemorrhages with minimal or absent signs of external trauma. It achieved worldwide recognition in the case of Louise Woodward, who was convicted of shaking 8-month-old Matthew Eappen to death in 1997 despite both sides agreeing that Matthew showed signs of direct head trauma so was, by definition, not a victim of SBS.

SBS was thought to be caused by the whiplash action of the child's relatively heavy head in association with weak neck muscles resulting in an acceleration-deceleration force sufficient to tear the bridging veins. The infant's head is made further susceptible to this type of injury by an immature, partially membranous skull, a relatively large subarachnoid space and a soft immature brain. However, the original studies had no scientific basis and were mainly hearsay and it now seems unlikely that such injuries can occur without some form of impact.

Visceral Injuries

The second most common cause of death from abuse is a ruptured liver. Other visceral injuries seen are ruptured spleen, pancreas and torn bowel—particularly the duodenum at its point of attachment. All these injuries require a huge amount of blunt force and cannot be explained by 'he fell off my lap'.

MISTAKEN DIAGNOSES

The following can mimic NAI and lead to a mistaken diagnosis:

- vitamin and mineral deficiencies, e.g. vitamins C (scurvy) and D (rickets), copper, calcium
- clotting abnormalities, e.g. haemophilia, von Willebrand's
- bone disorders, e.g. osteogenesis imperfecta
- pigment abnormalities, e.g. Mongolian blue spots (also known as slate grey naevi or dermal melanocytosis), birthmarks, striae
- alopecia areata can mimic hair pulling
- skin lesions, e.g. impetigo can look like cigarette burns
- self-inflicted injuries in older children
- injuries inflicted by siblings or other children
- accidental injuries.

THE CHILDREN ACT 1989

The *Children Act 1989* was implemented in October 1991 and it provided a fundamental change in child law in England and Wales. It has 108 sections and 15 schedules, with over 30 sets of Rules and Regulations. It is concerned with civil, not criminal, law and has two fundamental principles:

1. A child is best served by staying with the family of origin without recourse to legal proceedings.
2. If changes need to be made, any delay is bad for the child (Section 1(2)).

It makes the welfare of children paramount and recognises that children have rights and that their views must be respected in the appropriate circumstances. Section 1 states that no court orders will be made unless clearly in the best interests of the child and it outlines the following checklist that a court **must** consider in determining what a child's welfare demands:

1. The ascertainable wishes of the child—note that this is the first, although not necessarily the most crucial, decision.
2. Physical, emotional and educational needs.
3. Likely effect of any change in circumstances.
4. Age, sex, background and any other relevant characteristics.
5. Any current or potential harm to the child.
6. Capability of carer to meet the needs of the child.
7. The range of powers available to the court under the Act—the Act provides a choice of orders that are available to all courts and may be used in all types of proceedings.

There are four main ways in which issues affecting a child's future may be brought before a court:

1. **Wardship**—any individual can make a child a ward of court by issuing a summons, thereby ensuring that no decision affecting the life of the child may be made without leave of the court, e.g. withdrawal of treatment in a severely handicapped child. The *Children Act* restricted the powers of local authorities by not allowing them to make a child a ward of court without first bringing care proceedings.
2. **Divorce proceedings.**
3. **Private law applications**—e.g. contact orders for estranged grandparents.
4. **Care proceedings**—Local authorities had extensive powers in child welfare, but they were limited by the *Children Act*, which makes compulsory state intervention a last resort. A court can now only make a care order, placing a child under the supervision of the local authority if 'significant harm' can be demonstrated, this being defined as a 'deficit in or detriment to the standard of health, development and well-being'. The court must also be satisfied that a care order would be in the 'best interests' of the child and **better than no order at all**. This is the 'presumption of non-intervention' and has been considered by some to be the most important provision in the Act—the concept that a care order may not necessarily be the best way to protect the child's welfare.

The Act provides all courts with essentially the same powers and remedies and gives them timetables to reduce delay. Section 8 delivers a 'menu' of the orders available to the courts and these include:

- **Residence and custody orders**—these replaced the custody and access orders, respectively, which defined where and with whom the child would live or must be allowed to have contact. They have now both been replaced by the **Child arrangements order**, although they still apply.
- **Prohibited steps order**—this stops a person with parental responsibility from making certain decisions over the child's welfare without recourse to the courts.
- **Specific issue order**—this gives directions for dealing with a particular aspect of the child's care.

Applications for Section 8 orders are now regulated by the Child Arrangements Programme (CAP) and they cannot be used for 'looked after' children other than the residence order.

The Act promotes the idea of parental 'responsibility' rather than parental 'rights' and emphasises that this responsibility continues beyond divorce and when the child is in the care of a local authority, recommending the involvement of both parents in child protection conferences. It defines those who have 'parental responsibility':

1. The *mother and father* of a child if they were married at the time of the birth, even after divorce.
2. The *adoptive parents* of a legally adopted child.
3. The *mother* of a child born to unmarried parents, although the genetic father can gain it through a parental responsibility order, if agreed with the mother or by authority of the court.
4. A *guardian* as appointed through a will or court order.
5. Certain persons appointed through a care or residence order, e.g. a representative of the local authority.

Note that the Act allows anyone with parental responsibility to act alone, meaning that the consent of only one parent of a legitimate child is necessary. They may also authorise a third party to act on their behalf although they may not surrender responsibility. It allows anyone who has the care of a child to make decisions in the 'best interests' of the child so, for example, a teacher can give consent to a life-saving or life-preserving procedure.

The Act defines 'children in need' as being those who are:

1. Unlikely to achieve or maintain a reasonable standard of health or development or it will be impaired without the provision of services by a local authority.
2. Disabled.

It requires local authorities to:

- Identify such children and keep a voluntary register of all disabled children.

- Make assessments of the need.
- Provide appropriate services.
- Promote care within the family.
- Publicise services available.
- Ensure that families receive all relevant information.

Note that despite this increase in responsibilities for the local authorities, there has been no corresponding increase in resources.

The Act also brought in three new protection orders and it should be noted that the checklist discussed earlier does not apply to emergency proceedings (Table 14.2).

Finally, the Act also covers other areas such as provision of suitable accommodation, foster homes, child-minding and day care.

CHILDREN (SCOTLAND) ACT 1995

The *Children (Scotland) Act 1995* has many similar provisions to the *Children Act 1989* but child protection procedures in Scotland are different in that the system revolves around the Reporter to the Children's Panel.

The Reporter

This is a nationally appointed post and he considers reports from anyone with an interest in the welfare of a particular child. This can include teachers, social workers and the police. The Reporter must decide whether:

1. There are grounds for referral to a children's hearing. These include the commission of a criminal offence, lack of parental control and misuse of drugs or alcohol.
2. There is a need for compulsory measures of supervision—either in the home, with foster carers or in a Community home. 'Supervision' includes medical treatment, protection and control of a child.

TABLE 14.2
Protection Orders (PO)

	Emergency PO (EPO)	Police PO (PPO)	Child Assessment Order (CAO)
Duration	8 days—renewable once for a further 7 days	72 hours—not renewable	7 days—not renewable
Applicant	Anyone who then gains parental responsibility'—usually the local authority	Police Officer	Local authority
Apply to	Magistrates' court	None—Police Officer	Magistrates' court
Purpose	Prevent risk of serious harm by moving to or keeping in a place of safety. Replaced the 'place of safety' order	As EPO	To allow investigations and medical examination to prevent or assess risk of significant harm

If there are no grounds, then the Reporter either takes no action or refers the case to the local authority.

Children's Hearings

These are regulated by the *Children's Hearings (Scotland) Act 2011*, which has strengthened the rights of children within the hearings system and provided an advocacy system. They are legal tribunals, which are held in private and parents can accompany the child, unless they are named in the proceedings such as an NAI where the alleged perpetrator is the parent. The child may also bring a family friend or a professional such as a teacher. There is no legal representation. The Panel consists of three trained laypeople of mixed sex and varied background. The Reporter gives the 'statement of grounds' for referral and a decision is made on whether a compulsory supervision order is necessary. If the grounds are disputed, the case is referred to the Sheriff.

Children's Hearing Court Cases

At these hearings, the Reporter presents the case and protects the interests of the child. There may also be a safeguarder to represent the child and legal representation is allowed. The standard of proof is the civil standard, i.e. 'balance of probabilities' (see Chapter 2) and dress is informal, although evidence is given on oath. The Sheriff decides if the grounds are adequate. If they are, the case returns to the Children's hearing and if not, the referral is discharged.

Orders

The orders set out in the *Children (Scotland) Act* 1995 are similar to those in the *Children Act 1989* other than the Scottish equivalent of the EPO is the Child Protection Order (CPO) and application must be made to the Sheriff.

CHILD PROTECTION REGISTER

The Child Protection Register (CPR) has the following functions:

- Provide a confidential list of all children who have either been subjected to, or are thought to be at risk of, abuse.
- Provide statistical data.
- Assist in making the diagnosis of child abuse although it is important to note that it has limited value in this respect. If a child is not on the list, it does not mean that he is not being abused, it may simply mean that it has not yet been brought to the attention of the relevant authorities. However, the reverse may also be true—inclusion on the list does not automatically mean that he is being abused but it should raise suspicions.

It is maintained by the social services and it must be available 24 hours a day to relevant parties, e.g. emergency departments. To be included in the CPR, a child must be subject to a **Child Protection Plan** (CPP), which sets out how often social workers should check on the child, what changes are needed to protect the child and the level of family support required.

MAKING THE DIAGNOSIS

- Take a full history, making a note of any risk factors
- If a child confides that he has been abused, then you should:
  - Listen carefully
  - Reassure him that he is doing the right thing by telling you and that you believe him
  - Tell him that it is not his fault and he has done nothing wrong
  - Explain what will happen next
  - Report it to your Safeguarding Lead as soon as possible
  - Do **not** confront the abuser.
- Remember that physical abuse is often associated with other forms of abuse and that it can both recur and escalate. The aim is recognition and early intervention. This is particularly important in toddlers and infants who are at a greater risk of serious injury or death than older children.
- Fully undress and carefully examine the whole child if you have **any** suspicions.
- Plot the growth on a centile chart.
- Make legible, dated, contemporaneous, detailed notes with drawings of any injuries showing measurements.
- Check the CPR.
- Check for coagulation defects.
- Perform a skeletal survey if you have **any** suspicions.
- Get the paediatric teams and Child Protection Agencies involved **early**.

THE CHILDREN ACT IN PRACTICE

If you assess a child and believe them to be at 'significant risk' of harm, then your options are shown in Fig. 14.6.

SUMMARY

This chapter covers the distressing subject of child abuse. It outlines the legal structure of the specific types of crimes involved before defining the main categories of child abuse. It describes the different types of injuries

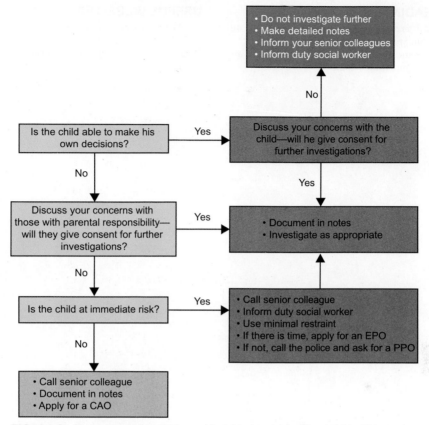

FIG. 14.6 Assessment of a child considered to be at 'significant risk' of harm. *CAO*, Child assessment order; *EPO*, emergency protection order; *PPO*, police protection order.

that classically occur in child abuse and provides warning signals in both the history and examination that should make the HCP suspicious that abuse is happening or that there is a high risk that it will occur. It takes the reader through the Children Acts of England, Wales and Scotland and highlights the various protection orders. It finally provides a useful flowchart on the options available to an HCP who sees or suspects child abuse.

CASE SCENARIOS

1. Danny is a 4-year-old boy with a painful and swollen left forearm who has been brought to the emergency department (ED) at midnight by his mother and she says that he fell over at about 2 p.m. Danny is quiet and does not make eye contact—are you concerned and what else do you want to know?
2. The mother says that she is a single carer for five children, all under 7. She has a new partner, but he does not live with them. She delayed attending because she

'had other things to do' and she 'thinks the neighbour may be looking after the other children'. On examination, you find old bruising to the pinna of his left ear, circular scars to his upper arms and an infected abrasion to his knee. You question his mother and she becomes defensive, saying that he is 'always falling over'. He is not on any medication, has no illnesses and she has not given him any analgesia. The X-ray shows a spiral fracture of his radius. Is this consistent with the story and what should you do now?
3. Danny's mother does not want to wait to see the paediatrician and tries to leave the department. What can you do?

See 'Answers to case scenarios'.

NOTE

1. Williams, R.A. Injuries in infants and small children resulting from witnessed and corroborated free falls. *J Trauma.* 1991;31:1350–1352.

FURTHER READING

Stark, M.M. *Clinical forensic medicine: a physician's guide*. 4th Edition. London: Springer; 2020.

Department of Education. *Children Act 1989 – Guidance and Regulations*. London: HMSO; 2021.

USEFUL WEBSITES

ECPAT UK: www.ecpat.org.uk/
NSPCC: www.nspcc.org.uk/
Scottish Children's Reporters Association: www.scra.gov.uk/

CHAPTER 15

The Sexual Offences Acts and Child Sexual Abuse

INTRODUCTION

The *Sexual Offences Act (SOA) 2003* of England and Wales came into force on 1 May 2004, repealing the *Sexual Offences Act 1956* and the *Indecency with Children Act 1960* and it applies to all offences committed on or after that date. It is the main legislation relating to child abuse and it created many new offences including causing a child to watch pornography, whether live or on video, assault by penetration and penetration of any part of a dead body. It was intended to improve on the preceding Acts by increasing maximum sentencing powers, extending the range of sentencing options and changing sentencing provisions. Section 74 of the Act also provided the first statutory definition of consent (see Chapter 5) as being **'he agrees by choice and has the freedom and capacity to make that choice'**. The corresponding legislation in Scotland is the *Sexual Offences (Scotland) Act 2009* and in Northern Ireland, it is the *Sexual Offences (Northern Ireland) Order 2008*.

SIGNIFICANT DATES

Prior to the enactment of the *SOA 2003*, there were other key changes in the law relating to sexual offences:

- **1960**—The maximum sentence for indecent assault on a woman increased from 2 to 5 years if the victim was under 13.

- **1985**—The maximum sentence for indecent assault on a woman increased to 10 years for any age and the maximum sentence for attempted rape increased from 7 years to life.

- **1993**—The presumption that a boy under the age of 14 was incapable of sexual intercourse and thus incapable of rape was abolished.

- **1994**—Nonconsensual anal intercourse was charged as rape rather than buggery, the maximum sentence for buggery on a boy under 16 increased to life and anal intercourse between consenting adults over the age of 18 was legalised.

- **1997**—The maximum sentence for offences against a child under 14 increased from 2 to 10 years.

- **1998**—The principle of 'doli incapax' was abolished by Section 34 of the *Crime and Disorder Act 1998*. This was the legal presumption that a child under 14 was incapable of knowing the difference between right and wrong and therefore lacked the capacity for intent to commit a crime, although it was rebuttable if a child were 10 to 13 and the prosecution could prove that the child was being more than 'naughty or mischievous'. This is also known as the 'age of criminal responsibility' and for England, Wales and Northern Ireland, it is now 10 although in Scotland it is 8, which is the youngest in Europe.

- **2001**—Section 1 of the *Indecency with Children Act 1960* was amended to increase the age of the victim from under 14 to under 16, so it broadened the scope.

- **2003**—Section 12 of the *Sexual Offences Act 1956* was omitted from the new *SOA*, which meant that it was no longer a criminal offence for homosexuals to participate in sex with more than one partner at a time. Part II of the new Act repealed the *Sexual Offenders Act 1997* and consolidated its provisions regarding registration of sex offenders and protective orders.

- **2019**—The *SOA 2003* was amended by the *Voyeurism (Offences) Act 2019* to make 'upskirting', which is the act of taking nonconsensual photographs under someone's skirt or kilt, an offence in England and Wales.

NONCONSENSUAL OFFENCES

Sections 1 to 4 of the *SOA 2003* deal with offences where the defendant has engaged in sexual activity with the complainant without the consent of the complainant (Table 15.1).

Section 1: Rape

Rape is defined as the intentional penetration of the vagina, anus and/or mouth by the penis, without either the consent or reasonable presumption of consent by the victim. This means that although the victim can now be of either sex, a woman can only be charged with rape as an accomplice. It is an indictable-only offence (see Chapter 1) and carries a maximum penalty of life imprisonment. Note that the previous definition of rape did not include oral penetration and if more than one orifice is penetrated, it should be charged separately. Being drunk is not an excuse—the victim does not have to be unconscious to be incapacitated by alcohol and/or drugs but it is up to the jury to decide on issues of consent and capacity. There is no onus on the victim to physically say or demonstrate that he does not give consent and consent is a continual process, so if the victim withdraws consent at any point, it becomes rape if the other party persists. If the victim receives injuries amounting to actual bodily harm (ABH) or worse (see Chapter 14), the defendant cannot rely on the 'rough sex' defence that his victim consented to the abuse as, under Section 71 of the *Domestic Abuse Act 2021*, a victim cannot consent to infliction of such a level of harm. As with all the nonconsensual offences, the prosecution must establish absence of consent and Sections 75 and 76 list ways in which lack of consent may be proved:

- Under Section 75, if the defendant did the relevant act as defined in Section 77 and he was aware that the following circumstances existed, the victim cannot be taken to have consented and the defendant could not have reasonably presumed that he had been given consent:
  - violence or threat of violence against the complainant or another person, e.g. a child
  - unlawful detention
  - complainant asleep or unconscious
  - complainant's physical disability
  - administering a substance to overpower or subdue, e.g. Rohypnol.
- Section 76 provides two further circumstances with the same provisos as earlier:
  - The defendant intentionally deceived the complainant as to the 'nature or purpose of the act'.
  - The defendant intentionally induced the complainant to consent by impersonating someone known to the complainant.

Note that while the circumstances described in Section 75 can be rebutted by defence showing that the complainant did consent, those in Section 76 cannot if proven.

Section 2: Assault by Penetration

This is a new offence created by the *SOA 2003* and as for rape, it is an indictable-only offence with a maximum penalty of life imprisonment. This offence can also be committed by females, as it involves nonconsensual penetration of the anus or vagina (but not mouth) by any part of the body, e.g. fingers, or an object, e.g. a bottle. This charge should be used instead of rape in cases where the victim cannot be sure if the perpetrator used the penis. The penetration must be 'sexual', as defined in Section 78 and shown in Box 15.1.

TABLE 15.1
Relevant Acts

Offence	Relevant Act
S 1: Rape	The defendant intentionally penetrating, with his penis, the vagina, anus or mouth of the complainant
S 2: Assault by penetration	The defendant intentionally penetrating, with a part of the body or anything else, the vagina or anus of the complainant, where the penetration is sexual
S 3: Sexual assault	The defendant intentionally touching the complainant, where the touching is sexual
S 4: Causing a person to engage in sexual activity without consent	The defendant intentionally causing the complainant to engage in an activity, where the activity is sexual

BOX 15.1
Definition of Sexual Penetration

Penetration, touching or any other activity is sexual if a reasonable person would consider that:

a. whatever its circumstances or any person's purpose in relation to it, it is because of its nature sexual, or

b. because of its nature it may be sexual and because of its circumstances or the purpose of any person in relation to it (or both) it is sexual.

Section 3: Sexual Assault

Sexual assault is an either way offence (see Chapter 1) and carries a maximum penalty of 10 years on indictment. It is defined as sexual (as defined under Section 78) touching of any part of the body with any part of the body or with anything else and case law has allowed this to include touching through clothing.

Section 4: Causing a Person to Engage in Sexual Activity Without Consent

This section has two parts:

- **Section 4—Nonpenetrative**. This is an either way offence and carries a maximum penalty of 10 years on indictment.
- **Section 4(4)—Penetrative**. This is an indictable-only offence and carries a maximum penalty of life imprisonment.

This offence can be committed on words alone, e.g. instructing the victim to masturbate themselves and it occurs in the following types of situation:

- The victim is forced to perform a sexual act on themselves.
- The victim is compelled to perform a sexual act with a third party, who may or may not give consent.
- The perpetrator makes the victim initiate the sexual activity.

This offence was created to allow female perpetrators exhibiting the same type of offending behaviour to be charged at a level equivalent to that of rape and also to cover a much wider range of sexual activities.

OFFENCES AGAINST CHILDREN

The *SOA 2003* classifies offences against children into three age categories: under 13, under 16 and under 18 years of age.

Sections 5 to 8: Offences Against Children Under 13

Note that although all these sections apply the same nonconsensual offences in Sections 1 to 4, consent is irrelevant in these cases as a child under 13 does not have the legal capacity to consent to sexual activity whatever the circumstances. There is also extensive overlap with Sections 9 to 13, which refer to children under 16, but Sections 5 to 8 were specifically created to allow offences against children under 13 to be subject to the same level of penalty without the child having to give evidence relating to consent. These are also offences of strict age liability—the prosecution only needs to prove the age of the child and that the relevant act occurred—and there is no defence of mistaken reasonable belief of the age of the victim.

- **Section 5: Rape of a child under 13.** This is defined as the intentional penetration of the mouth, anus or vagina of a child under 13 by the penis. It is an indictable-only offence with a maximum penalty of life imprisonment.
- **Section 6: Assault by penetration of a child under 13.** This makes the intentional penetration of the vagina or anus of a child under 13 with any part of the body or an object an offence. It is indictable only with a maximum penalty of life.
- **Section 7: Sexual assault of a child under 13.** Sexual touching of a child under 13 is an either-way offence with a maximum penalty of 14 years.
- **Section 8: Causing or inciting a child under 13 to engage in sexual activity.** As for Section 4, this creates two levels of offence—penetrative (indictable only with a maximum penalty of life) and nonpenetrative (either way with a maximum penalty of 14 years).

Sections 9 to 15: Offences Against Children Under 16

The *SOA 2003* provides that the age of consent to sexual activity is 16, so if the victim is under 16, any sexual activity is unlawful and the issue of consent is irrelevant. Sections 9 to 12 refer to adult defendants and Section 13 to juvenile defendants. Note that the defence of reasonable belief that the child was over 16 is available, unlike offences against children under 13.

- **Section 9: Sexual activity with a child.** This provides that the defendant must be under 18 and there must be sexual touching.
- **Section 10: Causing or inciting a child to engage in sexual activity.**

  Both sections create separate offences over whether there was penetration involved. If the assault was penetrative, the offence under Section 9 or 10 is indictable only with a maximum penalty of 14 years but if there was no penetration, the offence is either way, but the maximum penalty is still 14 years on indictment.
- **Section 11: Engaging in sexual activity in the presence of a child.** The child does not need to be aware that the activity is sexual but must be present, either in person or via a webcam.
- **Section 12: Causing a child to watch a sexual act.** The defendant over 18 causes a child to watch or look at pictures of a third person engaging in a sexual activity, i.e. pornography.
- Both sections are either way offences with a maximum penalty of 10 years on indictment.

- **Section 13: Child sex offences committed by children or young persons**. This section provides that if the defendant who committed the offences in Sections 9 to 12 is under 18, the maximum penalty on indictment will be 5 years.
- When considering whether to prosecute defendants under 18, the following should be considered:
  - Age, maturity and past experiences of the offender, e.g. was he coerced or subject to abuse himself?
  - Relative age and maturity of the parties and any previous relationship between them
  - Nature of the act
  - Any associated violence or threats.
- **Section 14: Arranging or facilitating commission of a child sex offence**. An example of this would be providing contraception to a child under 16. There is a defence available if the defendant can show that he did it to protect the child from pregnancy or infection, i.e. a child already in a consensual relationship, but not if the defendant intends harm, e.g. to offer the child for prostitution. The offence is either way with a maximum of 14 years on indictment.
- **Section 15: Meeting a child following sexual grooming**. The offence is committed if the defendant has intent to commit a sexual offence and meets the child, travels with the intention of meeting the child or the child travels with the intention of meeting the defendant. The child must be under 16, the defendant, who must be over 18, must be aware of that and there must have been previous communication, although it does not have to be sexual. The offence is either way with a maximum of 10 years on indictment.
- **Section 15A: Sexual communications with a child**. This is a relatively new offence, which was inserted by Section 67 of the *Serious Crime Act 2015* and makes it unlawful for an adult over 18 to communicate with a child under 16 in a sexual manner or conduct that encourages the child to respond in a sexual way, e.g. 'sexting'. The child does not need to respond and the method of communication is irrelevant, but the prosecution needs to show that it was done for the purposes of sexual gratification. The offence is either way with a maximum of 2 years on indictment and automatic registration as a sex offender.

Sections 16 to 27: Offences Against Children Under 18

- **Sections 16 to 24: Abuse of position of trust**. These provisions were created to protect children aged 16 to 17 who are believed to be vulnerable to abuse by those in a position of authority and/or trust. Their relationship with the abuser makes any ostensible consent void and positions of trust are defined in Sections 21 and 22, e.g. teachers, healthcare professionals (HCPs) and guardians. Sections 16 to 19 prohibit the same sexual behaviours as those described in Sections 9 to 12 and have the same distinction for charging and subsequent penalty if penetration occurred. Note that this is not an offence under Section 23 if the parties are legally married and the child is over 16.
- **Sections 25 to 27: Familial child sex offences**. These are similar offences but the person in the position of trust as defined in Section 27 is a family member, which can be anyone, including parents, siblings, step-parents, foster-parents or other relatives. The types of prohibited behaviour and the penalties are the same. Note that Sections 64 and 65 make it an offence to either commit or consent to penetrative sex with an adult relative, but these sections only relate to blood relatives and adoptive parents.

OFFENCES AGAINST PERSONS WITH MENTAL DISORDER

Sections 30 to 41 were inserted to protect those with a mental disorder that renders them vulnerable to sexual abuse and exploitation. Mental disorder is defined as 'any disorder or disability of mind' as per the *Mental Health Act 1983*, as amended by the *Mental Health Act 2007* (see Chapter 16), so it protects not only those with serious mental illnesses but also more chronic conditions such as dementia and learning disabilities. There are three categories of offence.

Sections 30 to 33: Offences Against a Person With a Mental Disorder Impeding Choice

The first category relates to the same sexual behaviours prohibited in Sections 9 to 12 (sexual activity with a child, causing or inciting a child to engage in sexual activity, engaging in sexual activity in front of the child or causing the child to watch a sexual act) but the word 'child' is substituted with 'person with a mental disorder impeding choice'. They also carry the same penalties. The prosecution must demonstrate that the defendant knew or could reasonably be expected to have known that the complainant had a mental disorder that would likely make him unable to refuse because:

a. he lacks the capacity to choose whether to agree to engaging in the activity, either because he lacks sufficient understanding of the nature or reasonably foreseeable consequences of the activity, or for any other reason, or

b. he is unable to communicate such a choice.

Sections 34 to 37: Offences Against a Person With a Mental Disorder by Using Inducement, Threat or Deception to Procure the Sexual Behaviour

The second category again relates to the same sexual behaviours as before but for these offences, the victim must have a mental disorder of such a degree that he has the capacity to refuse but is vulnerable to inducement, threat or deception to consent.

Sections 38 to 41: Offences by Care Workers Against a Person With a Mental Disorder

The third category is similar to the second, but the victim is persuaded to give consent through his familiarity with or dependence on the perpetrator. Note that medical evidence is usually required to establish the mental disorder, but if the defendant is a carer, there is a presumption that he would have known that the person had a mental disorder and it does not need to be proved. Section 42 provides the definition of what constitutes 'care' for these sections.

THE SEXUAL OFFENCES (SCOTLAND) ACT 2009

This Act is very similar to the *SOA 2003* in terms of its provisions and the groups that it was designed to protect but there are some striking differences:

- Prior to this Act, there was no statutory definition of rape in Scottish law and it was only defined in common law (see Chapter 1) as nonconsensual vaginal intercourse between a man and a woman, so male rape was excluded. This Act defines rape as penetration of the vagina, anus or mouth by a penis without consent, so it now applies equally to both sexes.
- There was also no statutory definition of consent, but this Act defines it as '**free agreement**'.
- The sexual offences are essentially the same but there are additional offences of 'sexual exposure' and 'administering a substance for sexual purposes'.
- The age of majority in Scotland is 16, so the descriptions of the age ranges are different. It refers to a 'young child' as one that is under 13 and there is still no defence of reasonable belief that the child was over 13. An 'older child' is one that is over 13

but under 16. The offences relating to 'abuse of trust' still apply to children (Section 18).

The penalties are stated in Schedule 2 and are comparable to those in the *SOA 2003*.

THE SEXUAL OFFENCES (NORTHERN IRELAND) ORDER 2008

This Act is essentially the same as the *SOA 2003* in that it has the same definition of consent and sexual offences. It was important in that it reduced the age of consent from 17 to 16 and it removed the duty of an HCP to report underage sexual activity in a child 13 to 15 where the other party is under 18, although they must still report children under 13 and consider any child protection issues. This means that HCPs can now treat children 13 to 16 without having to notify the police if it is done to:

- protect the child from sexually transmitted infections
- protect the physical safety of the child
- prevent the child from becoming pregnant
- promote the well-being of the child by providing advice.

CHILD SEXUAL ABUSE

The other types of child abuse are considered in Chapter 14, but the *SOA 2003* is the main legislation relating to child sexual abuse and exploitation, so it is discussed further here.

There are two types of sexual abuse:

1. **Contact**, e.g. rape, sexual touching, kissing, making a child undress and touch someone else
2. **Noncontact**, e.g. exposing a child to pornography or sexual acts, forcing a child to make, view or share indecent images.

The signs listed in Box 15.2 should make you suspicious that the child may be suffering sexual abuse.

BOX 15.2
Signs of Sexual Abuse

- Bed wetting and nightmares
- Fear of being alone or with strangers
- Using age inappropriate sexual words and knowledge of sexual behaviour
- Genital discharge, urinary tract infections, sexually transmitted diseases, pregnancy, unexplained injuries
- Drug and/or alcohol abuse
- Self-harm and other mental health problems
- Mood instability

BOX 15.3
Typical Vulnerabilities

- Dysfunctional home—parents with substance abuse or mental health issues, domestic violence, absent parents
- History of abuse of any sort
- Gang associations
- Recent bereavement or loss
- Peer pressure
- Learning disabilities
- Sexual orientation—either confusion or inability to discuss with family
- Homeless and 'looked after' children
- Low self-esteem
- Young carers

BOX 15.4
Signs of Exploitation

- Absent from home, care or school
- Physical injuries and change in appearance
- Repeated sexually transmitted diseases, urinary tract infections, pregnancy and terminations
- Unexplained funds, new clothes, jewellery or other items
- Drug and/or alcohol abuse
- Offending, especially drug dealing and stealing
- Mental health issues, including self-harm and suicide attempts
- New friends and estrangement from old friends and family
- Recruitment of others and gang membership

Although stranger abuse is not uncommon, children are most likely to be abused by someone they know, which could be their carer, family member, coach or teacher amongst others. This is why the *SOA 2003* has specific legislation about offences committed by a person in a position of trust. Both boys and girls are at risk of abuse but those most likely to suffer from sexual abuse and exploitation often share the typical vulnerabilities listed in Box 15.3.

These attributes also make these children more vulnerable to **grooming**, which is where the perpetrator develops an emotional relationship with the child to build trust so they can manipulate, abuse, traffic and exploit them. It is an offence under Section 15 of the *SOA 2003*. Groomers can be any sex, age or race and they may be known to the child or a stranger. The grooming can be for any length of time and it can be online, in person or both. The groomer may try to isolate the child and use blackmail to keep them in their thrall. Children rarely realise that they are being groomed and often have very complicated feelings about their groomer.

There is no specific offence of **child sexual exploitation (CSE)**, but sexual exploitation is defined in Section 51 of the *SOA 2003* as *'provision of sexual services, whether compelled to, for payment'*. This was amended by Section 176 of the *Policing and Crime Act 2017* to include 'streamed or otherwise transmitted' indecent child images to keep up with the changes in technology.

CSE occurs when a child is coerced into sexual activity in return for gifts, money, affection or status and children may be trafficked within or to the United Kingdom for this purpose (see Chapter 14). The coercion may also be in the form of violence or threats, either against the child or their friends and family leaving the child feeling that they have no choice but to comply. Child exploiters also use financial coercion by lending the child money that they can only repay by sexual favours. They are the same as groomers in that they can be any sex, age or race and they may also be 'recruiters', who are usually other CSE victims. CSE can be done online, in person or both, and children are often asked to send sexual images of themselves, which are then used to blackmail them into continuing. Children react to abuse in different ways, but Box 15.4 lists the classic signs that they are being exploited.

The provisions of Sections 47 to 50 of the *SOA 2003* are designed to try to protect children subject to abuse and CSE from being used in the sex industry ('child prostitution') and they all apply to children under 18:

- **Section 47**: Paying for the sexual services of a child. If there is penetration, it is indictable only with a maximum sentence of 14 years or life if the child is under 13
- **Section 48**: Causing or inciting CSE
- **Section 49**: Controlling a child in relation to CSE
- **Section 50**: Arranging or facilitating CSE. Sections 48 to 50 are all either way offences with a maximum sentence of 14 years on indictment.

Note that consent is not an issue, as they all relate to the perpetrator.

SUMMARY

This chapter covers the Sexual Offences Acts in England, Wales, Scotland and Northern Ireland and highlights the parts most relevant to healthcare professionals, with an overview of the important dates in the history of sexual offence law. It then provides a detailed description of child sexual abuse, with the different types and how to spot the signs that a child may be being abused and/or exploited.

FURTHER READING

Home Office. Strategy to end violence against women & girls: 2016-2020. July 2021. Available at www.gov.uk/government/publications/strategy-to-end-violence-against-women-and-girls-2016-to-2020.

Stark, M.M. *Clinical forensic medicine: a physician's guide*. 4th edn. London: Springer; 2020.

USEFUL WEBSITES

NSPCC: www.nspcc.org.uk/
ECPAT UK: www.ecpat.org.uk/
Faculty of Forensic and Legal Medicine: www.fflm.ac.uk

The Law Relating to Mental Health

INTRODUCTION

Despite the introduction of the *Mental Capacity Act 2005* and amendments by other acts, notably the *Mental Health Act 2007*, the *Mental Health Act 1983* remains the most important piece of legislation in mental health law, although its Scottish equivalent, the *Mental Health Act 1984 (Scotland)*, has been largely replaced by the *Mental Health (Care and Treatment) (Scotland) Act 2003*. Note that the Mental Health Acts apply equally to children as to adults, with the usual provisos regarding competence (see Chapter 5) and that the majority of patients who suffer from a mental disorder are treated and admitted to hospital informally and with their consent, without recourse to these Acts.

THE MENTAL HEALTH ACT (MHA) 1983

The *MHA 1983* replaced the *MHA 1959*, which in turn replaced the *Lunacy Act 1890* and its use is now regulated by the Care Quality Commission (CQC, see Chapter 7). It has 202 sections and is divided into 11 parts (1 repealed):

Part I: (Section 1): Defines mental disorder

Part II: (Sections 7–34): Compulsory admission to hospital and guardianship

Part III: (Sections 35–55): Remand to hospital through criminal proceedings

Part IV: (Sections 56–64): Consent to treatment

- **Part 4A:** Regulation of treatment of community patients not recalled to hospital—introduced by Section 35 of the *Mental Health Act 2007*
- **Part V:** (Sections 65–79): Mental health review tribunals
- **Part VI:** (Sections 80–92): Movement of patients around and in and out of England and Wales
- **Part VII:** (Sections 93–113): Regulation of the management of patient affairs and property—repealed by the *Mental Capacity Act 2005*
- **Part VIII:** (Sections 114–125): Duties of the local authorities and the Secretary of State
- **Part IX:** (Sections 126–130): Criminal offences such as forgery and ill treatment of patients

   Part X: (Sections 131–149): Miscellaneous matters such as the management of mentally ill patients in public places and the statutory protection of healthcare professionals (HCPs) from litigation for acts done in pursuance of the Act.

THE MHA 2007

This amended both the *Mental Health Act 1983* and the *Mental Capacity Act 2005* and was implemented in 2008. The most significant changes to the *MHA 1983* are the following:

- Redefinition of 'mental disorder' in Section 1 and removal of previous categories.
- Introduction of Supervised Community Treatment (SCT) and Community Treatment Orders (CTOs), which allow a patient who is not compliant with his medication in the community to be returned to hospital for compulsory treatment.
- Redefinition of the clinical professional roles, so there is now a much broader range of mental health professionals (MHPs) with the responsibility for treating patients without their consent.
- Creation of the role of 'approved clinician' (AC), who is a registered HCP (learning disability or mental health nurse, social worker, occupational therapist, psychologist or a doctor who specialises in mental health but is not on the GMC Specialist

Register for psychiatry) approved by the Secretary of State for the purposes of the MHA. There is also a 'responsible clinician' (RC), who has overall responsibility for a patient's care, including those under CTOs.

- Replacement of the 'approved social worker' (ASW) role with an 'approved mental health professional' (AMHP).
- 'Nearest relative' can now also be a civil partner and be displaced by the patient by application to the county court.
- Introduction of a new 'appropriate medical treatment' test as part of the criteria for continued detention under section and removal of the 'treatability' test. This means that a patient can now only be forcibly detained, or their detention extended if the correct medical treatment is available.
- Introduction of 'age appropriate services'—children under 18 years old admitted under the MHA must be held in an environment appropriate to their needs.
- Introduction of powers to reduce the time in which hospital managers must refer cases to the Mental Health Tribunal (MHT) and reduce the number of MHTs in England to 1.
- Introduction of new safeguards for patients receiving electroconvulsive therapy (ECT).
- Requirement for national authorities to provide independent medical advocates.

The changes to the *Mental Capacity Act 2005* are discussed in that section.

The *MHA 2007* also amended the *Domestic Violence, Crime and Victims Act 2004* to introduce new rights for victims of mentally disordered offenders who are not subject to restrictions.

In 2018 there were further amendments to the *MHA 1983* following the introduction of the *Mental Health Units (Use of Force) Act 2018*, which limited the force that could be used while restraining a patient and imposed training conditions and the use of body cameras by staff.

THE MHA AND CLINICAL PRACTICE
Section 1: Definition of Mental Disorder
Under the Act, **mental disorder** means any disorder or disability of the mind. This section is important, as a person must be suffering from a mental disorder as defined by the Act before compulsory admission to hospital or guardianship can be considered. Note that Section 2 provides that a person may not be considered to be suffering from a mental disorder simply because

they have a learning disability, unless that disability is associated with abnormally aggressive or seriously irresponsible conduct.

Section 2: Admission for Assessment
- **Duration:** Admission for assessment with or without medical treatment for 28 days or under.
- **Application:** Nearest relative (as defined in Section 26) or an AMHP approved under **Section 114** of the Act.
- **Recommendations:** Two doctors, one of whom must be 'approved' under Section 12(2) of the Act and the other (preferably) with previous acquaintance of the patient.
- **Grounds:** That the patient:
  1. is suffering from mental disorder of a nature of degree that warrants detention in hospital for assessment (and treatment) for at least a limited period, and
  2. ought to be so detained in the interests of his own health or safety or with a view to the protection of others.
- **Right of appeal:** Within 14 days of admission.
- **Discharge:** Nearest relative, managers or doctor but the doctor can bar discharge by the nearest relative. The patient must be discharged after 28 days unless he has been further detained under Section 3.

Note that if the patient is not sectioned or admitted informally following assessment, then under the Code of Practice, the AMHP and doctors must make arrangements for his further care. This is the most commonly used section.

Section 3: Admission for Treatment
- **Duration:** Admission for treatment **of a mental disorder** for ≤6 months unless the section is renewed under Section 20(4).
- **Application:** Nearest relative or an AMHP.
- **Recommendations:** Two doctors, one of whom must be Section 12 'approved'.
- **Grounds:** That the patient:
  1. is suffering from a known mental disorder of a nature or degree that makes it appropriate for him to receive treatment,
  2. there is appropriate medical treatment available and
  3. ought to be so detained and treated in the interests of his own health or safety or with a view to the protection of others.
- **Right of appeal:** Within the first 6 months and once during each subsequent period for which detention is renewed.

- **Discharge:** Nearest relative, managers or doctor but the doctor can bar discharge by the nearest relative.

This is used for patients where the diagnosis is already known.

Section 4: Application for Assessment in Cases of Emergency

- **Duration:** Admission for assessment only for 72 hours.
- **Application:** Nearest relative or an AMHP.
- **Recommendation:** One doctor who is only preferably acquainted with the patient. Once in hospital, it should be converted to a Section 2 or Section 3 and it should never be used simply for administrative convenience.
- **Grounds:**
  1. as for Section 2 and
  2. it is of urgent necessity to admit the patient and that admission under Section 2 would involve undesirable delay.
- **Discharge:** Automatic after 72 hours unless a second medical recommendation is given and received by the managers within that period.

Note that neither this nor the following sections allow for treatment without consent, but appropriate emergency treatment to contain the patient, e.g. sedation, may be given under common law in the best interests of the patient.

Section 5(2): Application in Respect of an Inpatient

- **Duration:** Detention of a patient already receiving **any form of inpatient treatment** for ≤72 hours, including any period during which a nurse's holding power was used. It cannot be used for outpatients or those attending the emergency department (ED).
- **Application:** The RC or his deputy, who must report to the managers on Form 12 that it appears that the patient presents a danger to himself or others and requires compulsory detention.
- **Discharge:** Automatic after 72 hours unless further powers have been taken under Section 2 or Section 3.
- **Right of appeal:** None.

Section 5(4): Nurses Holding Power

This applies to the same group of patients as Section 5(2) and it allows a mental health or learning disability nurse to detain a patient for up to 6 hours from the time that the decision is recorded on Form 13 until a doctor is found. The nurse himself must make the

decision and he cannot be instructed to invoke the section by anyone else. It must appear to the nurse:

1. That the patient is suffering from mental disorder to such a degree that it is necessary to immediately restrain him in the interests of his own health or safety or with a view to the protection of others.
2. It is not practicable to find or secure the immediate attendance of a doctor.

Note that the section is an emergency measure that lapses on the arrival of a doctor. The nurse must then complete Form 16 (Table 16.1).

Community care and treatment

Despite all the amendments, there are still no powers in the *MHA 1983* to forcibly treat patients in the community. Sections 7 and 8 set out the conditions for guardianship, which allow a patient to be required to live at a certain address or attend a specific clinic for treatment, but they cannot be enforced and the patient cannot be compelled to comply with the treatment. The only option is to apply CTOs to the patient under Section 17A at the time of discharge, which can then be used to return a noncompliant patient to hospital.

Section 12: Medical Recommendations

This grants approval from the Secretary of State to suitable doctors for the purposes of the Act and it recognises that the doctor has special experience in the diagnosis and treatment of mental disorders. Where two doctors are required, they should not normally be associated but two doctors from the same hospital can give the recommendations in cases of emergency.

Section 139

This prohibits proceedings against HCPs for any action related to the Act, unless it was done in bad faith or without due care. It means that civil actions may only be brought with the permission of the High Court and criminal proceedings must have the consent of the Director of Public Prosecutions. However, it is important to note that failure to apply the Act may also give rise to litigation.

THE MHA AND FORENSIC PRACTICE

The following sections apply to people who are believed to be suffering from a mental disorder and have been accused or found guilty of a criminal offence.

Section 35: Remand to Hospital for a Report

- **Purpose:** Allows a magistrate's court or Crown Court to remand an accused person who is either

TABLE 16.1
Summary of Main Sections of the Act Applicable in Clinical Practice

	Section 2	Section 3	Section 4	Section 5(2)	Section 5(4)
Type of application	Admission for assessment and treatment	Admission for treatment	Emergency admission for assessment	Detention of an inpatient	Nurses holding power
Application	Nearest relative or an AMHP	Nearest relative or an AMHP	Nearest relative or an AMHP	Report from doctor in charge of patient	None
Medical recommendations required	2, of whom ≥1 must be Section 12 approved	2, of whom ≥1 must be Section 12 approved	1, who should preferably know the patient	1, who should preferably know the patient	None
Length of detention	≤28 days	≤6 months	≤72 hours	≤72 hours	≤6 hours
Renewable?	Must convert to Section 3	Yes	Must convert to Section 3	Must convert to Section 3	Must convert to Section 3
Application to tribunal?	Within 14 days	Once in each 6-month period	No	No	No

AMHP, Approved mental health professional.

awaiting sentence or trial for an imprisonable offence, to a specified hospital for a report within 7 days.

- **Recommendation:** Either written or oral evidence from one doctor that the patient is suffering from a mental disorder and that it would not be practical to obtain a report on bail.
- **Duration:** Lasts 28 days and is renewable at 28-day intervals for up to 12 weeks by application to court, although the court can end the remand at any time.

If it becomes clear after the assessment that the prisoner requires treatment, it may be provided if he gives consent. If he refuses treatment, then the case must be returned to court in order to obtain a treatment order under Section 36, although the prisoner himself does not need to appear. Note that if the order came from a magistrate's court and the case is subsequently committed to the Crown Court, the order cannot be extended as the magistrate's court loses jurisdiction. Theoretically, this means that the patient must be either returned to custody or given bail, either of which may be very inappropriate for a mentally disordered patient. In practice, the patient is usually remanded to custody then immediately returned under Section 48 (see later).

Section 36: Remand to Hospital for Treatment

- **Purpose:** Allows a Crown Court only to remand an accused person who is awaiting trial for any

imprisonable offence except murder to hospital for appropriate medical treatment within 7 days. Note that this means that for cases still at the magistrate's court or where the charge is murder, there is no treatment order available preconviction unless the prisoner is then detained under Section 3 but both Section 35 and Section 36 are rarely used.

- **Recommendations:** Two and at least one must come from a Section 12 approved doctor.
- **Duration:** Lasts 28 days and is renewable at 28-day intervals for up to 12 weeks by application to court, but the court can terminate the remand at any time.

Section 37: Hospital and Guardianship Orders

- **Purpose:** Allows a magistrate's court or Crown Court to order hospital admission or reception into guardianship as an alternative to a prison sentence for prisoners found guilty of any imprisonable offence except murder. The prisoner must be admitted within 28 days.
- **Grounds:** As for Section 3.
- **Recommendations:** As for Section 36.
- **Duration:** Up to 6 months—renewable for a further 6 months then annually.
- **Right of appeal:** Not until the second 6-month period but it ceases to have effect if the prisoner appeals successfully against conviction.

Under Section 41, the Crown Court may add the restriction that the patient cannot leave or be transferred without the permission of the Home Secretary based on the oral evidence of one doctor that the patient presents a serious threat to public safety.

Sections 47 and 48: Transfer of Prisoners to Hospital

- **Purpose:** Allow the urgent transfer of prisoners suffering from a mental disorder to hospital on a warrant from the Home Office. Section 47 refers to sentenced prisoners; Section 48 to all others, including those on remand. It allows compulsory treatment to be given without consent.
- **Recommendations**: Both require two, one of which must be from a Section 12 approved doctor.
- **Duration**: No time limit.
- **Right of appeal**: Within the first 6 months.

The Home Secretary can restrict discharge under Section 49, which is applicable up to the expected date of release.

Section 135: Removing Patients to Hospital

If it is suspected that a person who is believed to be suffering from a mental disorder is being ill-treated, neglected or not properly controlled, or he lives alone and is unable to care for himself, the AMHP should be informed. He can request a magistrate's warrant to allow a police officer to enter the premises, by force if necessary, and remove that person to 'place of safety', which is usually the local psychiatric facility. The AMHP and a doctor must accompany the officer. The person can be detained up to 72 hours until a mental health assessment can be performed and another section applied, e.g. Section 2. Treatment can only be given with consent.

Section 136: Persons in Public Places

This authorises a police officer to remove a person that he believes to be suffering from a mental disorder from a public place to a 'place of safety' for up to 72 hours for assessment as earlier. The officer must believe that the person is in immediate need of care and control and/or presents a danger to himself and/or others. For this section, the 'place of safety' refers to a hospital (usually the local psychiatric facility), a police station, certain types of residential accommodation provided by the local authority or any other place deemed suitable by the police, including a private residence if the occupier agrees. Note that the CQC advises police to take the person to hospital[1] and the Code of Practice recommends that a local policy be agreed between the hospital(s), police and social services,

regarding the preferred places of safety and individual responsibilities.

For both Section 135 and Section 136, if the patient leaves, he can be retaken by the person last in charge of his custody, a police officer or the AMHP.

THE MHA AND CONSENT

Detention under the MHA does not necessarily mean that a patient is incapable of giving informed consent, but the Act provides that treatment can be given where the patient either lacks capacity (see Chapter 5) or refuses to give consent. Under Section 63, 'the consent of the patient shall not be required for any medical treatment given to him for the mental disorder from which he is suffering'. A detained person can be treated even if he refuses it and he may be restrained if necessary. However, any such treatment must be reasonable, i.e. in accordance with accepted medical practice (see Chapter 9) and the restraint should be sufficient only to allow the proposed procedure to be carried out. Although Section 63 refers to mental disorders only, it has been used to treat physical disorders where they are believed to either contribute towards, or be symptomatic of, the mental problem. This has included the force-feeding of people with anorexia, but it cannot be used where the physical problem is unconnected. In the case of *Re C* in 1993,[2] a schizophrenic with gangrene in his foot refused to consent to an amputation and he sought injunction to prevent it being done without his express consent. The judge ruled that he could refuse consent despite suffering from delusions, as he was capable of understanding what was proposed and the consequences of his refusal.

Note that a patient who is not capable of giving consent to his admission through reason of his mental disorder may still be admitted informally if he is admitted to an unlocked ward and does not attempt to leave or refuse treatment given in his 'best interests'. If such a patient then does attempt to leave and he is considered to be a danger to himself or others, he can then be detained under Section 5 of the MHA.

The following sections refer to specified treatments and are only applicable to patients detained under Section 3 or Section 37. The Second Opinion Appointed Doctor (SOAD) service is provided by the CQC to safeguard the rights of patients detained under the MHA who either refuse treatment or lack capacity.

Section 57: Treatment Requiring Consent and a Second Opinion

This applies to all patients undergoing:
1. any surgical operation for destroying brain tissue or its function
2. surgical implantation of hormones to reduce male sex drive.

Neither operation can proceed without:
1. informed consent from the patient
2. written certification from the SOAD that the patient has capacity and has given voluntary informed consent
3. written certification from the SOAD that the treatment is appropriate.

Section 58: Treatment Requiring Consent or a Second Opinion

This applies to administration of medicine for over 3 months and it can only be continued if:
1. the RC or the SOAD has certified that the patient has capacity and has given voluntary informed consent or
2. the SOAD has certified that the treatment is appropriate and should continue despite the patient either refusing to consent or lacking the capacity to consent.

Note that the patient has a statutory right under Section 60 to withdraw consent obtained under Section 57 or Section 58 at any time. This section no longer applies to ECT, which is now governed by Section 58A.

Section 62: Urgent Treatment

Treatment which is otherwise restricted by Section 57 and Section 58 may be given to a detained patient without either formal consent or a second opinion if it is deemed necessary to:
1. save the patient's life
2. prevent a serious deterioration in the patient's condition
3. prevent serious suffering
4. prevent the patient from becoming a hazard to himself or others.

Note that only treatment that is neither 'irreversible' nor 'hazardous' may be given in events 2–4 but the Act does not specify what treatment may or may not be used.

MENTAL HEALTH TRIBUNALS

These are independent bodies appointed by the Lord Chancellor. They consist of a psychiatrist and a lay member, and they are presided over by a barrister or, for Section 41 cases, a judge. They provide a right of appeal against detention or guardianship and the patient can apply for legal aid and be legally represented at the tribunal. Either the patient or the nearest relative can make applications and hospital managers or the Secretary of State may also refer patients.

MENTAL HEALTH (CARE AND TREATMENT) (SCOTLAND) ACT 2003

This Act is based on the 10 Millan principles:
1. Nondiscrimination—Patients suffering from a mental disorder should have the same rights and entitlements as any other patient if possible.
2. Equality—There should be no direct or indirect discrimination.
3. Respect for diversity.
4. Reciprocity—If the patient is obliged to comply with a programme of treatment and care, there is a parallel obligation on the health and social care authorities to provide appropriate services.
5. Care should be informal wherever possible.
6. Participation—Where they have the capacity to do so, patients must be fully involved in all aspects of their assessment, care, treatment and support. They must be given sufficient information in a format that they can understand and their wishes must be respected.
7. Respect for carers and their opinions.
8. Least restrictive alternative should be used wherever possible, taking into account the safety of others.
9. Benefit—Any intervention under the Act must be in the best interests of the patient.
10. Child welfare—This must be paramount in any interventions imposed on a child with a mental disorder.

Section 328 defines 'mental disorder' as any mental illness, personality disorder or learning disability, however caused or manifested and Section 328(2) specifically states that a person is not mentally disordered solely by reason of:
- sexual orientation
- sexual deviancy
- trans-sexualism
- transvestitism
- use of or dependence on drugs and/or alcohol
- exhibiting behaviour likely to harass, alarm or distress others
- acting as no prudent person would act.

The Act defines the form and functions of the Mental Welfare Commission (MWC) for Scotland and the MHT for Scotland. It also created the role of 'named person', which is similar to the 'nearest relative' of the English Act, and a series of detention certificates.

Section 36: Emergency Detention Certificate (EDC)

- This allows admission for assessment for 72 hours and is equivalent to the English Section 4.
- It can be granted by any registered medical practitioner but preferably with the consent of the mental health officer (MHO), who is equivalent to an AMHP.
- It does not authorise any treatment.
- An Approved Medical Practitioner (AMP) must review the patient within 72 hours. This is a doctor approved under Section 22, which is equivalent to the English Section 12. The AMP can suspend the EDC or impose a Short Term Detention Certificate (STDC), or the patient must be discharged after 72 hours.

Section 44: Short Term Detention Certificate (STDC)

- This allows admission for assessment with or without medical treatment for up to 28 days and is equivalent to the English Section 2.
- It can only be granted by an AMP and with the consent of the MHO.
- It allows compulsory treatment of a mental disorder and transfer to another hospital.
- The Responsible Medical Officer (RMO), who is the equivalent of the English RC, must inform the named person, the MHT and the MWC and also continually review the detention.
- It can be revoked by the MWC and the patient and named person can appeal to the MHT to have it revoked.
- It can be extended under Section 47.

Section 64: Compulsory Treatment Order (CTO)

- This is similar to the English Section 3 and allows treatment in hospital, but also in the community or at home for up to 6 months in the first instance, extendible for a further 6 months and then at yearly intervals.
- It is granted by the MHT after representations by the RMO, MHO, patient and their named person.
- There must be two medical reports, a report from the MHO and a proposed care plan, as it can only be granted if the appropriate medical care is available.
- The following compulsory measures can be authorised:
  - detention in hospital
  - administration of medication
  - imposing attendance at clinics or other community services to receive medication or other support
  - requiring the patient to reside at a certain address
  - requiring the patient to allow visits from the MHO or other care workers.
- The MHT may also grant an interim CTO, which allows all the same measures but for less than 6 months.
- CTOs must be reviewed by the RMO at least twice in the first 6 months.
- If a community patient is not compliant with their treatment under a CTO, they can be returned to hospital under Section 112.

Section 292: Removal From a Private Place

- This is equivalent to the English Section 135.

Section 297: Removal From a Public Place

- This is equivalent to the English Section 136.

Section 299: Nurses Power to Detain

- This is equivalent to the English Section 5(4) but it only lasts 3 hours, not 6.

WHEN TO APPLY THE MHA

- Section 2 or 44 should be used where:
  1. the diagnosis is not clear
  2. this is a first admission
  3. a thorough inpatient assessment is required.
- Section 3 or 64 should be used for patients:
  1. with a known diagnosis
  2. who have been assessed under Section 2 or Section 44 and have been found to require a further period of detention for treatment. Note that there is no need to wait for the 28 days to expire for applying for Section 3 or Section 64.
- Section 4 or 36 should only be used in genuine emergencies—not simply because it is difficult to obtain a second medical recommendation.

THE MENTAL CAPACITY ACT 2005

The *Mental Capacity Act (MCA) 2005* provides a framework for making decisions and acting on behalf of adults over 16 who lack capacity (see Chapter 5) and is equivalent to the *Adults with Incapacity Act (Scotland) 2000*. Section 1 outlines the five main principles underpinning the Act:

1. A person must be presumed to have capacity unless proved otherwise.
2. All practicable steps must be taken to assist the person to make their own decision before deciding on their behalf.
3. An unwise or irrational decision does not mean that the person lacks capacity.
4. Any decision taken on the behalf of someone who lacks capacity must be in their best interests.
5. Any decision made must be the least restrictive option available—this is particularly important when considering deprivation of liberty.

The Act also introduced other important provisions, including:

- A **Code of Practice** to assist people in following the Act.
- **Advance decisions** and the ability to plan ahead for future care (see Chapter 13).
- **Lasting Powers of Attorney (LPAs)**—These replaced the Enduring Powers of Attorney (EPAs) and they are appointed by someone with capacity to make financial and/or healthcare decisions on their behalf in the event of their losing capacity.
- Any decisions must be time, person and decision-specific, e.g. the decision to refuse a particular treatment may change with time and should be reviewed.
- The **Office of the Public Guardian (OPG)**— This administers the LPA system and also court-appointed deputies and guardians.
- The **Court of Protection (CoP)**—This has jurisdiction over the property, finances and welfare of people who lack capacity. It can appoint deputies to act on behalf of people who lack capacity, adjudicate on applications for deprivation of liberty and assist HCPs with more complex or difficult best interests decisions.
- The **Independent Mental Capacity Advocate (IMCA)** service to assist people who lack capacity and have no family members or friends to advocate on their behalf when making decisions in their best interests.
- It is now a specific crime to wilfully neglect a person who lacks capacity.

The *MCA 2005* was amended by the *MHA 2007* to introduce the **Deprivation of Liberty Safeguards (DoLs)**, which are procedures that authorise the deprivation of liberty of a person in a hospital or care home who lacks capacity, with the aim of protecting both the human rights of the individual and the carers from prosecution under the *Human Rights Act 1998*. Under the DoLS, the person being deprived of their liberty must be provided with a representative, the reasons for their detention and the right to appeal against the detention at the CoP. The *MCA 2005* was further amended in 2019 to add a new legal framework to replace the DoLS called the **Liberty Protection Safeguards (LPS)**. DoLS can only be used for adults over 18 but the new LPS will apply to people over 16 and to people in the community. They are also purported to be simpler to use but at the time of publication, the LPS have yet to come into force.

THE ADULTS WITH INCAPACITY ACT (SCOTLAND) 2000

The *Adults with Incapacity (Scotland) Act* is similar to the English *MCA 2005* in that it also provides a framework for making decisions for adults who lack capacity and there are five principles, but they are slightly different:

1. Any action taken must benefit the person.
2. The person should be encouraged and supported to make their own decision.
3. Any known wishes must be considered.
4. The decision must be the least restrictive option.
5. The wishes of anyone concerned with the person's welfare must also be considered, e.g. the named person, guardian or attorney.

Under the Act, those making decisions on behalf of someone who lacks capacity are regulated by the OPG (Scotland), the MWC (Scotland), the courts and local authorities. The main differences to the *MCA 2005* are the following:

- The court can appoint a **'Welfare Guardian'** to make decisions on behalf of people who lack capacity and they can also decide where the person should reside.
- LPAs are called **'Attorneys'** and the donor is the 'Granter'.
- The Act sets out the principles of providing medical treatment to people who are incapable of giving informed consent:
  - Emergency treatment can be given without recourse to the Act.
  - Nonurgent treatment can only be given once a doctor has assessed the patient as lacking capacity and completed a 'Section 47' certificate. This authorises treatment in the absence of consent, but it cannot be given forcibly or if the patient refuses.
  - The Welfare Guardian or Attorney can accept or refuse treatment on behalf of the patient but

the clinician in charge of the patient can ask the MWC to intervene if he does not consider it to be in the patient's best interests.

- As for the *MCA 2005*, some treatments require special safeguards, e.g. abortion, sterilisation and ECT. These require a second opinion under Section 48 or a court order.

SUMMARY

This chapter takes the reader through a detailed description of the most important pieces of legislation in mental health law and outlines the differences and similarities between the English and Scottish laws. It explains how the detention sections are applied depending on the circumstances and provides a practical guide to their correct use. It illustrates how the different acts can be used to protect people who lack capacity and how best to safeguard their human rights.

CASE SCENARIOS

1. Joan is a 90-year-old lady who is in hospital following a fall at home. Prior to this admission she had been living independently with support from her neighbours, but she was becoming more forgetful and confused and her personal care was poor. The fall has affected her mobility and the physiotherapist thinks she should be moved to a care home, but Joan wants to go back home. Her son lives over 100 miles away and thinks that Joan would be safer in a care home. Who decides what happens to Joan and what are the options? Who should be involved in the decision?
2. Joe has a long history of schizophrenia and cannabis use. He is found in the town centre being aggressive and abusive, so the police are called. What are their options?
3. Joe is taken to the nearest police station and is seen by the forensic medical examiner (FME), who finds that Joe is undergoing an acute psychotic episode and needs to be admitted for assessment and treatment. Joe refuses to go to hospital voluntarily so what can the FME do?

See 'Answers to case scenarios'.

NOTES

1. Care Quality Commission. A safer place to be, 2014.
2. *Re C (Adult: Refusal of treatment)* [1994] 1 All ER 819, (1993) 15 BMLR 77.

FURTHER READING

Medical Ethics Department. Mental Capacity Act toolkit. London: BMA; 2016.

Mental Health Act 1983: Code of Practice. London: TSO; 2015.

NHS Education for Scotland 2010. *Mental Health (Care and Treatment) (Scotland) Act 2003*.

The Law Relating to Alcohol and Driving

INTRODUCTION

Alcohol is the most commonly abused substance in the United Kingdom yet, unlike most other addictive drugs it is freely available. Crime statistics show that alcohol consumption is associated with criminal behaviour, particularly violent assaults and it is the cause of many serious road accidents. In 2018/2019, 1.3 million admissions to hospital were for problems related to alcohol, which was 7.4% of all admissions, but the healthcare profession has been notoriously poor at detecting and addressing these problems.

METABOLISM OF ALCOHOL

An alcohol is any substance that contains a hydroxyl group attached to a carbon atom and although there is no legal definition, it is usually considered to relate to one specific alcohol, ethanol. Some knowledge of the metabolism of alcohol is important, particularly in relation to the stages of acute and chronic alcoholism and to drink-driving offences.

Peak Alcohol Level

The blood alcohol level peaks at 30 to 90 minutes on an empty stomach, but it depends on the following (Fig. 17.1):
- Rate of absorption, as the elimination is very slow.
- Prior blood alcohol level.
- Duration of alcohol consumption—if the rate of consumption is low then the rates of absorption and elimination are similar and the peak is lower.

- Strength of alcohol—the optimum is 20%, as greater concentrations cause mucosal secretion and pyloric spasm and lower concentrations cause dilution, both of which delay absorption.
- Type of beverage—beer contains soluble nutrients, which delay absorption.
- Sex—for the same amount of alcohol, the peak level in women is higher as they have a higher fat:water index and alcohol is not distributed in fat.
- Body weight—the lower the weight, the higher the alcohol concentration as there is less body water to dilute it.
- Food in the stomach, which delays absorption.
- Physiological factors, e.g. gastric blood supply.
- Genetic variation, e.g. enzyme levels.
- Any condition that increases gastric emptying, as absorption is greatest in the duodenum, e.g. previous gastrectomy or drugs such as metoclopramide.

Elimination of Alcohol

The liver detoxifies 95% of alcohol, with 90% of the remainder being excreted by the kidney and the rest is eliminated in the breath and sweat. The rate of elimination in a normal person varies from 12 to 25 mg/100 mL of blood per hour, with an average of 15, which for a 70-kg man, corresponds to one unit per hour. In chronic alcoholics, this rate rises to up to 40 mg/100 mL/hour due to enzyme induction. Elimination is not linear and varies with the absolute level of blood alcohol, but 15 mg/100 mL/hour is usually a good estimate when attempting to back calculate blood or breath levels.

Having said that, there are so many variables to consider when attempting to back-calculate blood alcohol levels that it is rarely a useful exercise and it is usually reserved for more serious drink–drive cases where someone has died.

THE ACUTE EFFECTS OF ALCOHOL

Alcohol is a central nervous system depressant, affecting the highest centres first and the initial excitatory effects are caused by depression of the inhibitory centres. The effects are dose dependent, but there is huge interperson variation and chronic alcoholics develop

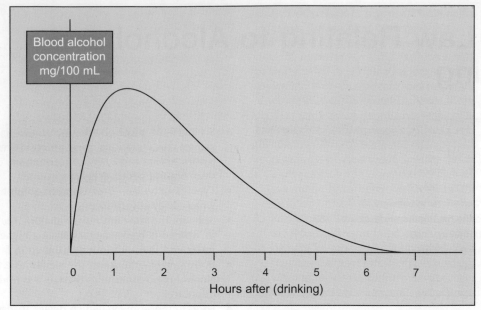

FIG. 17.1 Blood alcohol curve.

tolerance, so larger amounts must be consumed to achieve the same effects. There is a strong correlation between alcohol consumption and crime. In 2018 39% of all victims of violence said that their attacker was under the influence of alcohol and it is estimated that in 2017/2018, there were 561,000 incidents of alcohol-related violent crime[1] (Table 17.1).

THE CHRONIC EFFECTS OF ALCOHOL

There is a complex relationship between alcohol consumption and various diseases, but both the amount and frequency of alcohol consumption are important factors in the size and impact of the effect. Any research is complicated by the following:

- Except for violent deaths attributable to acute intoxication, the risks and benefits of alcohol consumption are likely to change with time.
- Quantitative assessment of drinking is generally based on self reporting, which may lead to misclassification.
- Alcohol consumption is usually associated with other lifestyle factors such as smoking or profession.
- Other constituents of alcoholic beverages may also affect the risks of disease.
- Drinking habits may change with age.

For overall mortality, the curve is U shaped, with an increase in all causes of mortality at higher levels of consumption. However, drinkers of small to moderate

TABLE 17.1	
Blood Alcohol Level and Behaviour	
mg/100 mL	**Effects**
<50	Not obvious, talkative, driving skills deteriorate
50–100	'Dizzy and delightful'—slurred speech, bravado, some loss of coordination
100–150	'Drunk and disorderly'—marked loss of coordination, staggering gait, disorientation
150–200	Nausea, noncooperative, loss of inhibition
200–300	'Dead drunk'—probable coma, vomiting, stupor, incontinence
300–400	Coma, impaired respiration, loss of reflexes
>400	'Devil's disciple'—dead

amounts of alcohol tend to have lower total mortality than nondrinkers, probably due to a fall in the risk of coronary heart disease. This cardioprotective effect seems to be mediated through an increase in the level of high-density lipoprotein (HDL) cholesterol, although there may also be other antiatherogenic and antithrombotic mechanisms. It is independent of sex and the type of alcoholic beverage. It is not known whether alcohol also reduces the relative risk of coronary heart disease in younger people, as most studies have been done in people over 40. Even if it does, other causes of alcohol-related death, especially accidents, are likely to outweigh any possible benefit given that the risk of cardiac-related death is lower anyway.

Other diseases are almost exclusively related to alcohol consumption such as cirrhosis and Wernicke's encephalopathy and alcohol has been shown to be a risk factor for various types of cancer, including cancer of the mouth, oesophagus, pharynx, larynx, liver and breast cancer in women.

Please see Box 17.1 for further hazards associated with chronic use of alcohol.

The current recommendations for maximum alcohol consumption are no more than 14 units (112 g ethanol) a week, spread over at least 3 days.

Alcohol misuse is common—in 2018/2019, there were an estimated 602,391 dependent drinkers in England alone,[2] with only 18% receiving treatment, but it is probably vastly underreported as healthcare professionals (HCPs) may not ask about alcohol intake and even if they do, the patient may not give a true approximate. This is compounded by the fact that many HCPs are unaware of the unit values for common alcoholic drinks and it is likely that the rate is now significantly higher in the wake of the COVID-19 pandemic and subsequent lockdowns (Table 17.2).

Most wine is 12% alcohol and a glass is 125 mL (six glasses to a bottle), so an average glass of wine contains 15 mL of alcohol, or 1½ units. When reading the table, be aware that super-strength beers and ciders contain much higher levels of alcohol—just one can of 330 mL extra-strong lager contains 4 units of alcohol. Also note that alcohol is less dense than water so volume per volume (v/v) alcohol content is not the same as weight per volume (w/v), e.g. 40% v/v whisky actually contains 32 mg of alcohol per 100 mL.

ALCOHOL AND THE HEALTHCARE PROFESSIONAL

In 1997, British Health Authorities were asked to consider the practicality of introducing compulsory liver function tests for all doctors every 2 years to pick up early warning signs of alcohol problems. This followed a fatal accident inquiry into the perioperative deaths of two patients where the surgeon subsequently admitted to having a serious drink problem. It was not instituted, partly because it was felt that it might still fail to identify the minority of those who are alcohol dependent, as liver function tests are not specific and may be normalised by a period of abstention. However, alcohol dependence is undoubtedly a problem amongst HCPs and the GMC, the NMC and the HCPC all advise that HCPs have an ethical obligation to disclose information about a colleague who is putting patients at risk. This also applies to patients who are misusing alcohol yet continue to drive or work in occupations that may put themselves or others at risk. The advice from the GMC and the Driving and Vehicle Licensing Agency (DVLA) is clear (see later), but HCPs often seem reluctant to follow it.

If the patient works in a hazardous occupation, you should encourage him to inform his employer that he is dependent on alcohol. If he refuses to do so, then you should ask for his consent for you to inform his employer on his behalf. If he refuses to consent, you still have a duty to inform his employer—preferably via the occupational health department. This is 'disclosure in the public interest' (see Chapter 6) but you must warn the patient that you intend to do so and confirm it in writing. The same advice applies if a patient is acutely intoxicated and you have reason to believe that he intends to drive. You have an ethical duty to inform the police, but again you must warn the patient that you intend to do so.

BOX 17.1
Hazards Associated With Alcoholism

1. Car accidents—either as a pedestrian or driver
2. Falls
3. Burns
4. Hypothermia
5. Susceptibility to infections
6. Liver, stomach and brain damage
7. Withdrawal fits

TABLE 17.2
Alcohol Content

Type	Percentage
Beer, lager and cider	2.5–4.5% v/v
Table wine	8–12% v/v
Fortified wines	20% v/v
Spirits	37–40% v/v
Liqueurs (and rum)	45% v/v or more

ALCOHOL AND DRIVING

In 2020, 220 people in the United Kingdom died in crashes where at least one driver was over the legal limit and there were an average of 12 crashes per day. At the legal limit, the chances of a serious accident are twice normal but at twice the legal limit, the risk is 20 times greater. Alcohol impairs vision, lengthens reaction time, reduces coordination and makes drivers think that they are invincible—a lethal combination. Driving while under the influence of drugs is also a problem—it causes 1:20 road deaths and showed a 110% increase from 5028 cases in 2018/2019 to 10,580 in 2020/2021. Both drug and drink drivers can be prosecuted under the *Road Traffic Act 1988* and it is illegal to drive if you are:

- unfit because you have taken alcohol or legal or illegal drugs
- over the prescribed limit of alcohol and/or drugs.

The following are the sections where the HCP may be involved.

Road Traffic Act 1988

Section 7(6): A person who, without reasonable excuse, fails to provide a specimen when required to do so in pursuance of this Section is guilty of an offence.

Section 4: Driving, or Being in a Charge, When Under Influence of Drink or Drugs

If a police officer suspects that someone who is driving, attempting to drive or in charge of a vehicle on a road or public place is impaired through alcohol and/or drugs, he can administer the following:

1. A roadside sample of either breath for alcohol (Breathalyser) or saliva ('Drugalyser') for drugs—currently cannabis and cocaine. If the breath test is over the prescribed limit and/or the saliva test is positive, the officer will arrest the suspect and take him to a police station.
2. Preliminary impairment tests under Section 6 (Field Impairment Tests), where the officer asks the suspect to complete a series of physical tasks such as standing on one leg and observes his ability to complete them. If the officer considers that there is evidence of impairment, he will arrest the suspect and take him to a police station. Note that if the saliva and/or breath tests are negative or below the limit, the officer can still arrest the suspect if he believes him to be impaired, as the blood samples taken at the station test for a much wider range of drugs.

Once at the station, a request will be made under Section 7 to provide a blood or urine sample, as for Section 5 next. The HCP may also be asked to assess the patient to exclude any underlying physical or mental illness or injury as the cause of the impairment (see Box 17.2).

The HCP must get informed consent (see Chapter 5), ensuring that the person is fully aware of the possible consequences, and write it in the notes. He must also tell the person that anything said during the assessment cannot be regarded as confidential and the examination must be meticulously performed and documented, as it is likely that the HCP will have to defend his opinions in court.

Note that there is now a separate Section 3A for causing death by careless driving when under the influence of drink or drugs, but it follows the same procedure as Section 4.

Section 5: Driving or Being in Charge of a Motor Vehicle With Alcohol Concentration Above the Prescribed Limit

The prescribed limits of alcohol for England, Wales and Northern Ireland are shown in the box, with the lower figures for Scotland in brackets (Table 17.3):

Random breath testing is not yet permissible in the UK despite being common practice abroad, but a person stopped for any reason may be tested at the discretion of the police officer. The roadside test is a screening procedure and if it proves negative, the person is allowed to proceed unless there are grounds for suspecting impairment due to drugs. If the driver refuses to perform the roadside test, then he will be arrested as **'failure to provide'** and taken to the police station to provide an 'evidential specimen for analysis'.

BOX 17.2
Conditions That May Result in Impairment

- Drug intoxication—both prescribed, e.g. benzodiazepines or antihistamines, and illicit, e.g. cannabis
- Drug and alcohol withdrawal
- Metabolic disorders, e.g. hypo- or hyperglycaemia, uraemia, porphyria, Addison's disease, thyrotoxicosis, hepatic failure
- Head injury
- Neurological disorders, e.g. Parkinson's disease, multiple sclerosis, epilepsy, vertigo, TIA
- High fever
- Cardiac disease, e.g. dysrhythmias
- Fatigue
- Carbon monoxide poisoning
- Mental illness, e.g. schizophrenia, hypomania

TIA, Transient ischaemic attack.

TABLE 17.3 Legal Limits	
	Legal Limits
Breath	35 (22) µg/100 mL breath
Blood	80 (50) mg/100 mL blood
Urine	107 (67) mg/100 mL urine

Note different units for breath.

BOX 17.3
Reasons for Failure to Provide a Breath Sample

- Asthma and other chronic lung problems
- Acute chest infection
- Injury to mouth, lip or face
- Tracheotomy, rib or chest injury
- Neurological problems, e.g. facial palsy
- Obesity
- Small stature
- Angina
- Neck problems, e.g. cervical spondylosis
- Comatose
- Inability to understand warning, e.g. mental disability
- Panic attacks and hyperventilation
- Alcohol intoxication (although this is *not* a 'reasonable excuse')

The roadside meter is set at 35 µg/100 mL breath and gives a green signal if the alcohol content of the breath is well below and yellow if it is near the threshold. If it shows a red signal, the driver will be arrested and taken to the police station for an evidential breath test.

Evidential breath samples are taken by a specially trained police officer (usually the custody sergeant) using an intoximeter. The accused must give two breath samples and the lowest reading is the one used. Although the legal limit is 35 µg/100 mL, no action is taken unless the reading is 40 or over. If the samples differ by more than a set limit ('unreliable sample') or if the intoximeter is not available, then the sergeant can require a blood or urine sample, with the type of sample being at his discretion. If the accused does not give a sample without reasonable excuse (see Box 17.3), then he will be charged with **'failure to provide'**, although the HCP may be consulted as to whether the accused has provided a 'reasonable excuse'.

If the accused is in hospital following an accident, the evidential sample must be of blood and the ED staff may be asked to take it, but it cannot be taken by anyone involved in the clinical care of the patient. Under **Section 9**, the police are obliged to notify the clinician in charge before requiring the patient to provide a sample. If the clinician objects, the requirement cannot be made but the objection must be on the basis that it would be 'prejudicial to the proper care and treatment of the patient' to either provide the sample or be given the obligatory warning that he or she will be prosecuted for **'failure to provide'**.

If the accused is able to give informed consent (see Chapter 5), the HCP must get specific consent and write it in the notes, ensuring that the patient is fully aware of the possible legal consequences. He must be very clear that this is **not** a therapeutic procedure and note that poor comprehension due to intoxication is not a valid excuse. Any swabs used *must* be alcohol-free. If the patient is unconscious or otherwise unable to give informed consent, the HCP can be asked to take an evidential sample of blood without consent under **Section 7A**, if the officer believes:

1. he has grounds to request a sample under Section 7
2. the suspect was involved in an accident
3. the suspect is or may be unable to give informed consent for valid medical reasons.

Note that the sample taken in such circumstances cannot be tested until the person from whom it was taken has:

1. been informed when and where it was taken
2. been required to give his permission for a laboratory test of the sample
3. given his permission.

If he refuses to give permission without reasonable cause, he will be charged with **'failure to provide'**. Please remember that blood taken for diagnostic purposes cannot be subjected to analysis under the *Road Traffic Act* 1988.

Whether in hospital or in custody, the HCP decides the site of venepuncture and is allowed three attempts to take one sample, which is then divided into two equal parts and labelled. The accused has the option to have one part tested at his own expense at an independent laboratory from an approved list.

If the accused refuses to give blood without the grounds shown in the Box 17.4, then he is charged with **'failure to provide'**.

If the accused cannot provide a blood sample, the police can request a urine sample, which are collected by the police officer. The accused is asked to empty his bladder, then the urine that he produces is collected over the next hour *under the supervision* of the police officer. The process is degrading and open to contamination, so it is avoided wherever possible. If the accused cannot or will not provide a urine sample, then he is charged with **'failure to provide'**, unless there is a medical reason as shown in Box 17.5.

Note that if the defence depends on a 'reasonable excuse' based on medical grounds for failure to provide any of the evidential samples—breath, blood or urine, they must provide the prosecution with that evidence prior to the court case so the prosecution can seek an expert medical opinion, as the burden of proof is then on the prosecution to negate it. The court must then consider:

1. The medical evidence of mental or physical inability to provide the specimen, and
2. If there is a causal link between that condition and the failure to provide the specimen.

Section 5A: Driving or Being in Charge of a Motor Vehicle With Concentration of Specified Controlled Drug Above Specified Limit

This is a summary only offence (see Chapter 1), which came into force in 2015 to bring the offence of drug driving in line with that of drink driving and avoid the need to prove associated impairment. **Section 11** defines a 'controlled drug' in the same way as Section 2 of the *Misuse of Drugs Act 1971*, i.e. any substance or product specified in Parts I, II or III of Schedule 2 of the *Misuse of Drugs Act 1971* (see Chapter 18). If the drug is found in the blood or urine at a level *above*

the specified limit, it is an automatic charge, *unless* the drug has been prescribed and dispensed in accordance with the *Misuse of Drugs Act 1971* and taken according to medical advice, although the suspect can still be charged under s 4 if his driving was impaired as a result. In the case of poly-drug use, there should be separate charges for each drug. Although the section states blood or urine, there are currently no specified limits set for urine, so the specimen must be of blood. There are currently 17 drugs with stated levels listed in the *Drug Driving (Specified Limits) (England and Wales) Regulations 2014* and the *Drug Driving (Specified Limits) (England and Wales) (Amendment) Regulations 2015*. The levels have been set using figures from a panel of experts to account for such factors as "accidental exposure" meaning that this is not a 'zero tolerance' offence. Drugs are classified into illegal (zero tolerance so only accidental exposure levels) and legal (legal so a risk-based approach) (Table 17.4):

TABLE 17.4
Prescribed Limits for Illegal and Legal Drugs

	Threshold Limit in Blood
ILLEGAL	
Benzoylecgonine	50 µg/L
Cocaine	10 µg/L
Delta-9-tetrahydrocannibinol (cannabis)	2 µg/L
Ketamine	20 µg/L
Lysergic acid diethylamide (LSD)	1 µg/L
Methylamphetamine	10 µg/L
Ecstasy or 3,4-methyl enedioxymethamphetamine (MDMA)	10 µg/L
Heroin	5 µg/L
LEGAL	
Amphetamine	250 µg/L
Clonazepam	50 µg/L
Diazepam	550 µg/L
Flunitrazepam	300 µg/L
Lorazepam	100 µg/L
Methadone	500 µg/L
Morphine	80 µg/L
Oxazepam	300 µg/L
Temazepam	1000 µg/L

MEDICAL ASPECTS OF FITNESS TO DRIVE

Each time an HCP writes a prescription, he should also consider the fact that different drugs can affect fitness to drive and advise the patient accordingly. Prescribed drugs with a known impact on driving are listed in Box 17.6.

Licensing requirements depend on the type of vehicle given, but an ordinary license is valid up to the age of 70 then it must be renewed every 3 years, but

---

BOX 17.6
Drugs Affecting Ability to Drive

- Prescribed, e.g. tranquillisers, antiepileptics, antidepressants, antipsychotics, antihistamines, analgesics, anaesthetics
- Illicit, e.g. opiates, cannabis, lysergic acid diethylamide (LSD)

TABLE 17.5
Conditions Affecting Driving on an Ordinary License

Disease	Driving Restrictions
Epilepsy	Fit-free for ≥1 year
Narcolepsy	Yearly medical review once controlled
Chronic neurological disease, e.g. Parkinson's, MS	None if medical assessment confirms no impairment
CVA, TIA	Stop ≥4/52 then start if no residual disability
Vertigo, Meniere's	Stop until symptoms controlled
Benign brain tumours	Stop for 1 year then 3-yearly review
Head injury	Stop 6/12–1 year
Angina	Stop if rest pain or on driving
Myocardial infarction/CABG	Stop ≥4/52
Arrhythmias	Stop if disabling or distracting
Syncope	Stop until cause identified and controlled
Hypertension	None unless drugs cause problems
Heart valve disease/HOCM	None
Heart/lung transplant	None
DIABETES	
Insulin dependent	Cannot drive light goods or small passenger-carrying vehicles
Non-insulin dependent	None
VISION	
Acuity	At least 6/12
Fields	At least 120° on the horizontal meridian with no significant field defect within 20° of fixation
Colour blindness	None
Deafness	None
MENTAL ILLNESS	
Psychosis	Stop until medical assessment
Depression	None unless suicidal
Schizophrenia	None if controlled
Dementia	Stop until medical assessment
DRUGS	
Opiates	Stop for 1 year then screening
Cannabis	Stop for 6/12 then screening

CABG, Coronary artery bypass grafting; *CVA*, cerebrovascular accident; *HOCM*, hypertrophic obstructive cardiomyopathy; *MS*, multiple sclerosis; *TIA*, transient ischaemic attack.

this is automatic unless the driver reports a problem. A photocard license must be updated every 10 years from the age of 50 and every license states that a driver has a legal duty to:

- Inform the DVLA of any potential or actual medical disability that may affect his driving.
- Respond fully and accurately to any requests for information from the either the DVLA or HCPs.
- Comply with the requirements of the issued license, including any medical reviews mandated by the DVLA.

HCPs have a duty to:

- Inform patients about the impact of their condition and/or medication on their safe driving ability
- Remind the patient that he has a legal duty to inform the DVLA of any relevant condition
- If the patient cannot or refuses to do so and continues to drive, inform the DVLA themselves and it is best practice to write to the patient, confirming that this has been done.

For medical standards, there are two groups of drivers and the standards are significantly higher for Group 2:

- Group 1—includes cars and motorcycles
- Group 2—includes large lorries (category C) and buses (category D).

In the United Kingdom, the DVLA provides guidelines for HCPs called *Assessing fitness to drive—a guide for medical professionals* and some of the medical conditions affecting driving with an ordinary license are shown in Table 17.5.

SUMMARY

Alcohol is one of the most addictive substances and yet it remains freely available despite multiple studies showing a close correlation between alcohol, violent crime and road deaths. This chapter covers all aspects of alcohol from its metabolism and acute and chronic effects to the latest drink and drug drive legislation. It highlights those sections where the healthcare professional may become involved by either taking samples or assessing for other causes of impairment to drive. It also covers medical assessment of fitness to drive and the relevant advice from the DVLA.

CASE SCENARIOS

1. A man has been brought into the ED following a car accident in which he was the driver. His car was badly

damaged, but he apparently has only minor injuries and his breath smells of alcohol. You are in charge of the care of this patient and a police officer approaches you to ask if he can request a blood sample from this man, as he is suspected of driving while under the influence of alcohol. Do you give permission?
2. The officer tells you that your patient was driving erratically but slowly before mounting the pavement and hitting a bollard. An open bottle of whisky was found in the car. You decide to give permission but ask to assess the patents' capacity to consent to the sample before allowing it to taken. Do you need to do this and what would you need to ascertain to reassure yourself that the patient does have capacity?
3. You decide that the patient has capacity and he agrees to provide the sample. The officer asks you to take it. Do you do so and if not, to whom can you delegate the task?

See 'Answers to case scenarios'.

NOTES
1. The nature of violent crime in England and Wales: year ending March 2018. ONS 2019.
2. Burton, R. et al. *The public health burden of alcohol and the effectiveness and cost-effectiveness of alcohol control policies: an evidence review.* London: PHE; 2016.

FURTHER READING
Stark, M.M. *Clinical forensic medicine: a physician's guide.* 4th edn. London: Springer; 2020.
Payne-James, J., Jones, R.M. *Simpsons forensic medicine.* 14th edn. Boca Raton: CRC Press; 2019.
Driver and Vehicle Licensing Agency. Assessing fitness to drive—a guide for medical professionals, 2021.

USEFUL WEBSITES

DVLA: www.gov.uk/government/organisations/driver-and-vehicle-licensing-agency

CHAPTER 18

The Law Relating to Drugs

INTRODUCTION

Writing a prescription is potentially one of the health-care professional's (HCP) most hazardous tasks. From overprescribing tablets to someone who later uses them to commit suicide to the patient who forges or changes your prescription, the whole process can be fraught with difficulty. Even if your prescription is perfect, you are still supplying a poison, albeit with the best of intentions, to a patient who neither would nor could have it without your intervention. It is therefore vital for every HCP to have a sound knowledge of both the pharmacology and the legislation surrounding drugs. There are already many excellent pharmacology books so this chapter will concentrate on the legal side.

PRESCRIBING

Guidance on the prescription of different classes of drugs can be found in the British National Formulary (BNF), the Nurse Prescribers' Formulary (NPF) and in Medicines, Ethics and Practice: A Guide for Pharmacists.

Prescribing was restricted to doctors and dentists until 1992, when the *Medicinal Products: Prescription by Nurses Act 1992* and subsequent amendments to the *Pharmaceutical Services Regulations* allowed registered nurses, midwives and health visitors to become nurse prescribers. There are now three types of nurse prescribers:

1. **Community practitioner nurse prescribers (CPNP)**—these are nurses who have successfully completed a Nursing and Midwifery Council (NMC)-registered CPNP course and are registered as such with the NMC. They can only prescribe from the NPF for Community Practitioners, which contains dressings, appliances, general sales lists (GSL) drugs and 13 prescription-only medicines (POM) (see later).

2. **Independent prescribers (IP)**—these are practitioners who have successfully completed a registered IP course and are registered as such with their professional body. They are responsible for the assessment and treatment of patients with both diagnosed and undiagnosed conditions and for making prescribing decisions. They can prescribe any medicines, including all products and medicines listed in the BNF, unlicensed medicines (not in Scotland) and all controlled drugs in Schedules 2–5, but only where it is clinically appropriate and within their field of competence. They can prescribe cocaine, dipipanone or diamorphine for organic disease but not for the treatment of addiction.

3. **Supplementary prescribers (SP)**—these are practitioners who have successfully completed the supplementary part of the prescribing course and are registered as such. They can prescribe within an agreed patient-specific clinical management plan (CMP), agreed in partnership with a doctor or dentist.

If they have completed the relevant SP or IP course and registered as such with their own regulatory body, other allied HCPs, including pharmacists, paramedics and physiotherapists can now be SPs or IPs too.

Please see Box 18.1 for the correct way in which a standard prescription should be written. Note that if the prescription is for a controlled drug, it must be handwritten, signed and dated. It is then valid for 28 days. It must state both the patient's and the prescriber's names and addresses. The total quantity of the preparation or the number of dosage units must be written in words and figures.

Prescriptions are usually written for one particular patient but there is a special type of prescription called 'patient group directions' (PGD). These were previously known as group protocols and they provide a legal framework for HCPs to supply and/or administer a named medicine or vaccine in a known clinical situation where the patients may not be identified prior to

---

BOX 18.1
A Prescription Should

- Clearly identify the patient for whom it is intended
- Be given, where possible, with the patient's informed consent
- Be clearly written, typed or computer-generated and indelible
- Clearly identify the substance by either its generic or brand name and state the preparation, strength, dose, frequency and route of administration, timing, start and finish dates
- Record the weight of the patient where the dose is weight-dependent
- Be signed by the prescriber
- NOT be a substance to which the patient is known to have an adverse or allergic reaction
- Only be given over the telephone if not previously prescribed in certain circumstances

---

arrival, e.g. group vaccinations at school or in a baby clinic. They must be drawn up by a local senior doctor or dentist and a pharmacist and signed by both of them.

DISPENSING

Any HCP can legally dispense drugs, but the patient has a right to expect that it will be done with the same expertise as a qualified pharmacist, so it should only be done under very rigid guidelines, if at all.

ADMINISTRATION

Any HCP who administers a drug must:

- Know the therapeutic use, normal dose, side effects, precautions and contraindications of the drug that they are giving
- Ensure that it is the correct patient
- Ensure it is the correct prescription
- Check the dose, route of administration and timing
- Check any calculations necessary with a second HCP
- Ensure that there are no contraindications, especially allergies and coexisting treatment
- Check the expiry date
- Clearly, contemporaneously and accurately record the time, dose and route of administration
- Never prepare intravenous injections in advance or give an injection prepared by another HCP unless they are present.

- Clearly, contemporaneously and accurately record if the drug is not given and the reason, e.g. patient refusal
- Note and act upon any adverse reactions.

MEDICATION ERRORS

In 2020, the *British Medical Journal* reported that an estimated 237 million medication errors were made every year in England, costing the NHS over £98 million and resulting in the deaths of more than 1700 people. The NHS National Reporting and Learning System (NRLS—see Chapter 7) defines a patient safety incident (PSI) as 'any unintended or unexpected incident, which could have or did lead to harm for one or more patients receiving NHS care'. Medication errors are PSIs where there has been an error in:

- prescribing
- preparing
- dispensing
- administering
- monitoring
- providing advice on medications.
  They can be errors of either:
1. commission, e.g. incorrect dose or drug
2. omission, e.g. failure to monitor anticoagulant therapy or a missed dose.

   All medication error PSIs should be reported to the NRLS and HCPs are advised to speak to their indemnity provider at the earliest opportunity.

MEDICINES AND HEALTHCARE PRODUCTS REGULATORY AGENCY

The Medicines and Healthcare products Regulatory Agency (MHRA) was established in 2003 as the executive Agency of the Department of Health & Social Care and it is responsible for ensuring the safety and efficacy of all medicines and healthcare devices in the United Kingdom. It runs the **Yellow Card** scheme in conjunction with the Commission on Human Medicines (CHM) and this is the method by which HCPs, coroners and pharmacists (and patients and carers) can report any adverse drug reactions (ADRs). They are asked to report **any** possible ADRs in 'new' drugs, i.e. those that are marked with an inverted black triangle (▼) in the BNF and any **serious** reaction in 'older' established drugs. Yellow Cards are assessed to establish whether there is a causal relationship between the drug and the ADR and if there are any possible risk factors that might increase the chance of the patient developing a reaction, such as age or concurrent disease.

The risk of a newly identified ADR is then evaluated in the context of the efficacy of the drug, its known side effects, the target population, the condition it is used to treat and other drugs in the same class. The action then taken depends on the gravity of the reaction, but outcomes include:

1. The new side effect is listed in the product information.
2. Use of the drug is changed to maximise the benefit and minimise the risk, such as changes to the dose or preparation, or it may be restricted to more serious conditions.
3. Special warnings may be issued.
4. The drug may be withdrawn if the risk of harm is considered to outweigh the benefit.

ADDICTION AND DRUG DEPENDENCE

In 2018/2019, there were 2917 deaths from drug misuse and it was the reason for over 18,000 hospital admissions.[1] In the same period, 1 in 11 adults had taken drugs, with 1 in 25 using Class A drugs[2] and the most commonly used drugs were cannabis, cocaine and nitrous oxide. Men have a higher rate of drug use and dependence than women, but women are more susceptible to cravings and more prone to relapse. Addiction to prescription drugs is also a growing problem in the United Kingdom and is currently under review. Box 18.2 shows a list of commonly misused prescription drugs.

Dependence Syndrome

This is defined as compulsion to use drugs with an overriding focus on drug-seeking behaviour plus one or more of the following:

BOX 18.2
Commonly Misused Drugs

- Benzodiazepines, e.g. diazepam (Valium), temazepam
- Opioids, e.g. diamorphine (heroin), morphine, pethidine, dihydrocodeine (DF118), buprenorphine (Temgesic)
- Cannabis, e.g. 'weed', resin cakes, reefers
- Cocaine and crack
- Ecstasy (MDMA), e.g. 'e'
- Amphetamines
- LSD and mescaline
- Volatile substances, e.g. glue, aerosols, solvents, petrol

---

1. Tolerance—the amount of drug needed to give the desired effect rises.
2. Withdrawal—both physical and psychological symptoms occur on stopping the use.
3. Use of drugs to relieve or avoid withdrawal symptoms.

Addiction in HCPs

HCPs are at particular risk of becoming addicted, as they do highly stressful jobs and have unique access to supplies. The very nature of their roles means that their addiction poses a particular risk to the public and while most recovering addicts can continue to work, an HCP may need to be removed from their environment in order to limit their access to the drugs. Also, HCPs often find it more difficult to admit to their addiction and to get an effective, confidential treatment that will not jeopardise their future careers.

Addicted HCPs usually come to notice in a crisis situation such as stealing drugs or being found intoxicated. An internal investigation then follows which is frequently a protracted and inefficient method of dealing with what is essentially a medical problem. Treatment is often challenging, as the HCP may find the role of the patient difficult in itself without the associated high expectations of compliance and recovery. Return to work is possible under strict supervision to protect both the HCP and the public and there are now more resources available—addicted doctors and dentists can self-refer to NHS Practitioner Health (see 'useful websites' at the end of this chapter), the Royal College of Nursing (RCN) provides support for nurses and the College of Paramedics have a range of services for paramedics. In the United States, testing for drug and alcohol use in the workplace is routinely employed and it has been instituted in Britain for jobs in which safety is critical. A review of the law suggests that employers in such situations are entitled to test for and enforce strict policies on drug and alcohol use, provided that this has been made explicit in the contract, and that a positive test can be the basis of dismissal.

LEGISLATION
Medicines Act 1968

This was passed in response to the Thalidomide disaster with the aim of preventing any further such injuries. Thalidomide was a drug used to relieve morning sickness in early pregnancy, but it proved to have catastrophic teratogenic side effects. The *Medicines Act 1968* provides a legal framework for the manufacture, licensing, prescription, supply, labelling, packaging and administration of 'medicinal products', defined as being made or supplied solely for administration to an animal or human for a 'medicinal purpose'. A 'medicinal purpose' is diagnosing, treating or preventing disease, induction of anaesthesia, contraception or any other permanent or temporary effect on physiological function, so it covers a huge number of different products. The *Medicines Act 1968* also:

- established the Medicines Control Agency (now part of the MHRA), the Committee on Safety of Medicines (now the CHM) and the British Pharmacopoeia
- controls advertising and sales
- classifies medicines into the categories shown in Box 18.3.

Unlicensed Medicines

These have no product licence and no manufacturer liability. If they are given to a patient, the prescriber carries full liability and they should only be given on a patient-specific prescription where there is no licensed alternative available.

Poisons Act 1972

This defines a poison as 'any substance that has a harmful effect on a living system'. It covers all **non-medicinal** poisons and divides them into two parts:

1. **Part 1**: These can only be sold by a retail pharmacist, e.g. strychnine, oxalic acid, phenols.

> ### BOX 18.3
> ### Categories of Medicines
>
> **PRESCRIPTION-ONLY MEDICINES (POMs)**
> - These may only be supplied or administered to a patient on the instruction of a doctor, dentist or independent prescriber (IP).
>
> **PHARMACY-ONLY MEDICINES (P)**
> - These may only be bought from a registered primary care pharmacy, under the supervision of a pharmacist.
>
> **GENERAL SALE LIST MEDICINES (GSLs)**
> - This is a very limited list subject to various limitations and can be bought from any retail outlet. It includes all veterinary, herbal and aromatherapy products and also paracetamol, aspirin and cold products.

---

2. **Part 2**: These can also be sold by a person on the Local Authority list, e.g. an ironmonger. These include sulphuric acid, paraquat and formaldehyde.

The purchaser must provide his name, address and the purpose for which the poison is intended.

Misuse of Drugs Act 1971

This Act repealed the *Drugs (Prevention of Misuse) Act 1964* and the *Dangerous Drugs Acts 1965* and *1967*. It prohibits the possession, supply and manufacture of drugs and other products unless it has been legalised under the *Misuse of Drugs Regulations 1985* (see later). Storage of controlled drugs comes under the *Misuse of Drugs (Safe Custody) Regulations 1973*. Please note that all controlled drugs must be kept in a locked receptacle and a car is not regarded as such unless they are further locked within a bag or in the boot of the car.

The Act applies in Northern Ireland, England, Scotland and Wales and it has 40 sections and 6 schedules, although the following are of most relevance to the HCP:

- **Section 1**—this established the **Advisory Council on the Misuse of Drugs**, which is responsible for a national surveillance of which drugs are being misused, what constitutes misuse and whether the use of a particular drug causes sufficient harmful effects to have a widespread social impact. If it does, the Council must inform Parliament of the steps necessary to control the problem. They also advise on rehabilitation, treatment facilities and public education.
- **Section 2**—this section divides controlled drugs into the three categories shown in Box 18.4. These categories determine the penalties for illegal possession and supply, but the Act allows the category of a drug to be changed and for it to be released from control as new evidence appears (Table 18.1).
- **Sections 3, 4 and 5**—these control the import and export, supply, destruction, possession and trafficking of controlled drugs.
- **Section 6**—this prohibits the cultivation of cannabis plants.
- **Section 7**—this defines the exemptions granted by the Home Office to allow certain people to possess specific controlled drugs.
- The Act also allows the police or 'other authorised person' to enter the premises of anyone producing or supplying drugs, inspect any relevant documentation and search anyone that they have 'reasonable grounds' to suspect may be carrying controlled drugs. This search also extends to their vehicle.

BOX 18.4
Categories of Drugs

Class A: e.g. heroin, morphine, cocaine, crack, opium, pethidine, LSD, methadone, mescaline, methamphetamine

Class B: e.g. oral amphetamines, cannabis, codeine, dihydrocodeine, ecstasy, barbiturates, ketamine, GBH, GBL

Class C: e.g. anabolic steroids, benzodiazepines, khat

TABLE 18.1
Maximum Penalties

	Possession	Supply and Production
Class A	7 years/unlimited fine/both	Life/unlimited fine/both
Class B	5 years/unlimited fine/both	14 years/unlimited fine/both
Class C	2 years/unlimited fine/both	14 years/unlimited fine/both

- Under the Act, a doctor can be prevented from prescribing, administering or supplying controlled drugs if he:
  1. Fails to notify an addict under the *Misuse of Drugs (Notification and Supply to Addicts) Regulations 1973* or treats an addict with heroin or cocaine for anything other than the organic disease (Section 13).
  2. Is found guilty of an offence under the Act (Section 12).
  3. Has had his practice limited by the General Medical Council (GMC) (see Chapter 10), e.g. for irresponsible prescribing.
- **Section 14**—if a doctor is prohibited under the Act, he can appeal to a **tribunal** of five people, which include doctors and lawyers. The hearing is private and the doctor can be legally represented. If this procedure fails, then the doctor can appeal to an **advisory body**, whose decision is final.
- **Section 15**—if a doctor's practice is considered to be dangerous and worthy of rapid restriction, the case can be referred to a **professional panel**, where again the doctor can be legally represented. The panel can issue a temporary direction, which prohibits the doctor from prescribing or supplying controlled drugs for 6 weeks, although this is

subject to 28-day extensions until he appears before the tribunal.

Misuse of Drugs Regulations 1985

These are divided into schedules that allow different classes of people to possess and supply controlled drugs:

Schedule 1—this lists drugs with no accepted therapeutic value and defines those people who are licensed to supply, administer and possess them, usually for research purposes. It includes cannabis, ecstasy, lysergic acid diethylamide (LSD) and mescaline.

Schedules 2 and 3—these list >100 drugs that may be administered and supplied by doctors, dentists, vets and IPs to patients who may only then legally possess them. A patient can only obtain the prescription from one prescriber and it must be for his own use. The majority of the drugs are not in common use and those that are used are labelled 'CD' in the BNF. Schedule 2 drugs include methadone, morphine, cocaine, dihydrocodeine, pethidine, Ritalin and amphetamines. Schedule 3 drugs are subject to prescribing restrictions and include flunitrazepam (Rohypnol), barbiturates, temazepam and buprenorphine. These schedules also specify how a prescription for a controlled drug should be written (see earlier).

Schedule 4—this has two parts:
  I. Most minor tranquillisers, including the benzodiazepines (not flunitrazepam or temazepam)
  II. Anabolic steroids—the medicinal form can be possessed without a prescription but not supplied.

Schedule 5—this exempts certain preparations containing small amounts of controlled drugs from rigid control, so there is no prohibition of import, export, possession or supply of such drugs. Examples include codeine and pholcodine linctus and codeine phosphate tablets.

The Act also defines the layout and entry-keeping of the registers that must be kept for drugs in schedules 1 and 2.

Psychoactive Substances Act 2016

This regulates and restricts the sale, production and supply of psychoactive substances, which are defined as anything that stimulates or depresses the central nervous system and so alters the person's mental or physical state. They are also known as 'legal highs'. The Act bans all psychoactive substances but then excludes alcohol, caffeine, tobacco and other nicotine-based products, any medicinal products and all drugs regulated by the *Misuse of Drugs Act 1971*.

HANDLING ILLEGAL DRUGS

You are not required by law to remove suspicious packages from patients and if you do remove illegal drugs and then return them to the patient or a relative, you are supplying drugs and you could be **liable to prosecution**. The drugs should be either handed to a police officer or destroyed, although if you do destroy the drugs, you could be charged with obstruction if the police are involved. Note that if it is a schedule 1 drug and you remove it, then you are committing an offence simply by possessing it. If you are forced to handle illicit drugs, e.g. the patient is unconscious, ensure that all your actions are witnessed and that you make witnessed contemporaneous notes. If the patient has a legally prescribed controlled drug such as methadone, it must be stored in the controlled drugs cupboard. It can then be either administered or restored to the patient on discharge.

Suspects may also transport drugs in various body cavities ('body packers' or 'mules') or swallow drugs when arrested ('body stuffers' or 'swallowers') and the HCP may be asked to remove the drugs. In a conscious patient, this should only be done with informed consent and the patient must be made fully aware of the possible consequences of massive drug ingestion. If the patient is not able to give consent, then the HCP must act in the 'best interests' of the patient. Note that under Section 55 of the *Police and Criminal Evidence Act 1984*, the police can ask the HCP to perform an intimate search without consent and this is covered in Chapter 4.

SUMMARY

This chapter covers everything that a healthcare professional (HCP) needs to know about both legal and illegal drugs. It provides detailed information about the right way to write a prescription and the correct procedure to follow when preparing and administering medication. It outlines what constitutes a drug error and what to do if it happens. The chapter defines drug addiction and dependence and highlights why this is a particular problem for HCPs—both for their patients and themselves—and gives the HCP sources of help and advice. It then goes through all the relevant legislation before offering advice on dealing with handling illegal drugs.

NOTES

1. See www.digital.nhs.uk/data-and-information/publications/statistical/statistics-on-drug-misuse/2019.
2. Home Office. Drugs misuse: findings from the 2018/19 Crime Survey for England & Wales. Statistical Bulletin 21/19. 2019.

FURTHER READING

British National Formulary.
Nurse Prescribers Formulary.

USEFUL WEBSITES

Yellow Card scheme: www.yellowcard.mhra.gov.uk/
NHS Practitioner Health: www.practitionerhealth.nhs.uk/
Royal College of Nursing: www.rcn.org.uk/
College of Paramedics: www.collegeofparamedics.co.uk/

Answers to Case Scenarios

CHAPTER 3—PREPARING A POLICE STATEMENT

1. Hammer blows cause lacerations with surrounding bruising and are often associated with an underlying transverse fracture of the ulna if this was a typical defence injury. Your patient does not have any signs of these types of injuries and superficial incised wounds are seen more commonly in self-harm or in attempts to fabricate a story of assault, so the story is not consistent with the injuries. Self-inflicted injuries are usually found on the nondominant side of the body, so it is important to ask if your patient is right- or left-handed, and there is often scarring from previous attempts, so you should also check for that.

2. Although stab wounds are classically deeper than they are wide, which is the opposite to slash wounds, they are both types of incised wounds, so although unlikely, this is possible.

3. You must have the consent to release of the medical information by the patient. If you have any 'dates to avoid' such as holidays or exam dates, ensure that you complete them on the back of your statement.

4. Unless they have asked you to attend on a day that you have previously informed them that you will not be available, you must attend. You are appearing as a professional witness, so there is no need for representation by your indemnity provider and they would have no authority to do so.

5. You are not appearing as an expert witness in this case, so you should not guess or venture any opinions that you cannot back up with evidence, qualifications in the field of injury causation and/or experience. You can say that the injuries were consistent with those caused by a sharp object, but you should not conjecture as to the type of weapon or whether it was self-inflicted, even if that is what you believe. NEVER go beyond the limits of your expertise or qualifications and give short answers wherever possible.

CHAPTER 4—FORENSIC SAMPLES

1. You should always ask for the circumstances in any situation where you have been asked to take samples, as you may be able to advise the officer on the most appropriate types of sample, e.g. if the victim bit or scratched the accused during the assault, then it would be essential to swab the wounds and document the injuries. Timing of the assault is also important, as if it happened a week ago, there would be no evidential advantage to taking the swabs and it is technically assault to take samples in such circumstances. If there is any doubt about the date or time, take the samples as there is unlikely to be another opportunity.

2. As the boy is 16, you must get consent from both the boy and the appropriate adult, who must also be present during the sampling. You should also ideally have a male chaperone present if both you and the appropriate adult are female. You must assess the capacity to consent for both the boy and the appropriate adult and ensure that they both understand that it is not a therapeutic examination and the potential consequences of both providing samples and refusing to consent.

3. If this is a second suspect from the same case of alleged rape, you must decline due to Locard's Principle—every contact leaves a trace, which means that there is a high risk of cross-contamination with the first suspect via you. The second suspect must be examined and sampled by a different healthcare professional (HCP) at a different location.

CHAPTER 5—CONSENT

1. You must assess whether she has the capacity to consent to antibiotic treatment:
   a. Does she have sufficient maturity to provide you with an adequate medical history, especially with regard to the possibility of previous allergies and is she able to understand the benefits and risks of taking, refusing or not taking the full course of the antibiotics?
   b. Can she retain the information that you have given her?
   c. Can she weigh up that information and use it to come to an informed decision?
   d. Can she communicate that decision to you?
   If you are satisfied that all the above criteria can be met and that Alice is not under any duress so her

consent is both informed and voluntary, then you can give her the antibiotics. If you are not satisfied, you should encourage Alice to return with someone with parental responsibility. If she refuses, then you must base your final decision on her primary welfare and best interests. Remember that Section 5 of the *Mental Capacity Act 2005* authorises healthcare professionals to act in the patient's best interests in order to preserve life or prevent deterioration in their health. In all eventualities, remember to record your decisions and reasonings accurately and contemporaneously.

2. Although you considered on the last occasion that Alice had the capacity at that time to consent to treatment, this is now a very different situation because:
   a. The level of capacity needed to refuse treatment has been established in law to be higher than that to be able to consent to treatment.
   b. Alice is under the influence of drugs and alcohol, so her capacity is temporarily reduced.
   c. She has voluntarily returned to your clinic despite apparently not wanting treatment.
   Given these factors, you would be justified in initiating emergency, life-saving treatment without her consent, although you should make every effort to persuade her to give consent and you should also try to contact someone with parental responsibility. Again, you must record your decisions and reasonings accurately and contemporaneously.

CHAPTER 6—CONFIDENTIALITY AND DISCLOSURE

1. There are limited circumstances in which you are legally obliged to disclose medical information to the police:
   a. Under the *Road Traffic Act 1988*, you must disclose the name and address of a person who has attended for treatment of an injury that may have been received during the commission of a road traffic offence, if requested to do so by the police. You should not disclose any clinical information without the patient's consent, unless directed to do so by the Court.
   b. Under the *Terrorism Act 2000* and the *Terrorism Prevention and Investigation Measures Act 2011*, you must disclose any information that may prevent the commission of an act of terrorism or lead to the apprehension, prosecution or conviction of a suspected terrorist.

   c. All wounds inflicted by a gunshot or sharp instrument must be reported to the police unless they are the result of an accident or self-inflicted. No other personal or clinical information should be shared at the time of reporting the incident.
   Where possible or appropriate, you should attempt to gain the consent of the patient prior to the disclosure but only if it would be safe to do so. Always try to ascertain the reason for the request; the limits of the information required and the legal authority for the request. Keep your disclosure within the limits of the request and provide only the relevant and necessary clinical information.

2. You must disclose the information if ordered to do so by a judge, but you can make representations about the amount and type of information that you release if you consider it unnecessary to the scope of the request.

3. You should try to persuade him to warn Jane and advise him that he has a moral obligation to do so. He should also tell her to attend the clinic so she can be tested too.

4. You should contact Jon at the earliest opportunity and confirm that Jane is not aware of his HIV status. If he has not told her, you must advise him that if he is not prepared to tell Jane now that they will no longer be practising safe sex, you will. This is an example of disclosure in the public interest, as Jane's need to know this information outweighs Jon's right to confidentiality. You must still give him the opportunity to consent to the release of the information—either by telling her himself or allowing you to do so.

CHAPTER 13—EUTHANASIA, WITHDRAWING TREATMENT AND ADVANCE DECISIONS

1. An Advance Decision (AD)-declining life-sustaining treatment must be signed and witnessed and you cannot assume that this was just an error, as he may have changed his mind so you should start life-saving measures. You must also attempt to get more information.

2. An unsigned AD has no validity to refuse treatment, so you must continue to act in the best interests of the patient. Although it seems clear that he did not want to be put on a ventilator, it is not stated on the AD and you do not know if the situation has changed in the last 5 years, so you should continue treatment.

3. Although it is more difficult to stop treatment than to continue, you should not ventilate this patient, although you can and should make him as comfortable as possible through any other measures short of ventilation. This version of his AD is compliant with the terms of the *Mental Capacity Act 2005* and you must respect the wishes expressed in it, even if you do not agree with them.

CHAPTER 14—CHILD ABUSE AND THE CHILDREN ACTS

1. Young children are often shy with strangers and Danny is probably also in pain so his behaviour is not unusual, but the 10-hour delay between the injury and the presentation should be questioned. You should also ask about the home situation to check for any risk factors for child abuse and any indicators in Danny's past medical history such as previous injuries, prematurity and underlying illnesses.

2. Spiral fractures are associated with torsion, traction or angulation not direct impact, so this injury is not consistent with 'falling over' and Danny has other older injuries, which are pathognomonic of abuse. There are also other multiple risk factors evident in the history, including parental attitude, change in home situation, delay in reporting and multiple injuries of differing ages. This is all highly suggestive of child abuse and you should refer him to the Child Safeguarding Lead in your department. Danny should also have a full skeletal survey completed and clotting disorders should be excluded. You must ensure that the Child Protection Agencies have been alerted and check the Child Protection Register.

3. Danny appears to be at risk of immediate harm, so you should call the police so that they can apply for a Police Protection Order.

CHAPTER 16—THE LAW RELATING TO MENTAL HEALTH

1. It should be assumed that Joan has the capacity to decide where she would live unless proven otherwise, so her capacity should be formally assessed. It should be noted that her capacity may fluctuate given the history of confusion and forgetfulness, so her capacity may need to be reassessed for each decision made. She must be given all the relevant information to reach that decision in a way that she can understand, including the potential challenges of returning home and the risks. If she is found to have capacity but is not fit to go home immediately, she should be moved to a rehab facility to assess her needs and if she could go home with a suitable care package in place. Her son should be consulted but made aware that it is ultimately his mother's decision and the physiotherapist should also be asked for their opinion. If Joan lacks capacity, then the decision should be made in her best interests.

2. The police can arrest him for public disorder, but given his history, it would be more appropriate to detain Joe under Section 136 of the *Mental Health Act 1983* or Section 297 of the *Mental Health (Care and Treatment) (Scotland) Act 2003* and remove him to a place of safety. Ideally, this should be the local psychiatric facility, but it is often the police station or emergency department (ED).

3. The forensic medical examiner (FME) should contact the approved mental health professional (AMHP) and ask for a formal mental health assessment at the station. The AMHP will then contact the on-call psychiatrists, arrange for an assessment and check the hospital bed status. Once Joe has been seen by the AMHP and the psychiatrists, at least one of which must be Section 12 approved, a decision will be made about Joe's future management. If he still refuses to go voluntarily and he remains a danger to himself and/or others, then he must be placed under either Section 2 or Section 4 of the *Mental Health Act 1983*. As Joe already has an established diagnosis of schizophrenia, it would be more appropriate to admit him under Section 4.

CHAPTER 17—THE LAW RELATING TO ALCOHOL AND DRIVING

1. Unless you have any concerns that it might adversely affect your patient to either provide the specimen of blood or be given the statutory warning that failure to provide the sample would render him liable to prosecution, you have no grounds to refuse. However, you should ask for the circumstances of the accident, as this may help you decide if your patient has occult injuries.

2. Although the sample can be taken without consent under Section 7A of the *Road Traffic Act 1988*, this procedure is only rarely used and usually reserved for cases where the patient is unconscious. It is best practice to assess capacity and ask for informed consent to give the sample, as failure to provide the

specimen is also an offence under Section 7(6) of the *Road Traffic Act 1988*. When assessing capacity, you must ensure:

a. The patient understands the venepuncture procedure and the potential consequences of both providing and refusing to provide the sample.

b. He can retain that information.

c. He can use it to make a decision.

d. That he can communicate the decision to you by any means. Note that for this procedure, he must also communicate with the police officer and demonstrate to him that he understands the whole process and consequences.

3. As the person in charge of the care of the patient, you cannot legally take the sample and must delegate it to someone else not involved in the care of the patient. It can be taken by anyone skilled in phlebotomy—it does not have to be a doctor or nurse—but if the sample comes back over the limit, it is very likely that the person who takes the sample will have to complete a statement and may have to attend court, so it is preferable to ask someone senior.

Legislation Covering Legal Aspects of Medicine

Chapter	Subject	Related Legislation (UK Unless Stated Otherwise)
1	Criminal law	*Prosecution of Offenders Act 1985*
	Statute interpretation	*Interpretation Act 1978*
	District judges	*Access to Justice Act 1999*
	Youth Court	*Criminal Justice Act 1991*
	Crown Court	*Courts Act 1971*
2	Crown Prosecution Service	*Prosecution of Offences Act 1995*
	Arrest and prosecution	*Police and Criminal Evidence Act (PACE) 1984*
	Disclosure of evidence	*Criminal Procedure and Investigations act 1996* *Criminal Procedure (Scotland) Act 1995*
	Expert witness role	*Civil Procedure Rules 1998*
3	Statements in criminal cases	*Criminal Justice Act 1967* (Section 9) *Magistrates Courts Act 1980* (Section 102) *Magistrates Courts Rules 1981* (Rule 90)
	Statement on behalf of someone else (documentary hearsay)	*Criminal Justice Act 1988*
4	Forensic samples (collection)	*Police and Criminal Evidence Act (PACE) 1984* *Prisoners and Criminal Proceedings (Scotland) Act 1993* *Road Traffic Act 1988*
	Intimate searches	*Misuse of Drugs Act 1971* *Police and Criminal Evidence Act (PACE) 1984*
5	Consent to procedure	*Human Fertilisation and Embryology Act 1990*
	Tutor-dative	*Adults with Incapacity (Scotland) Act 2000*
	Consent and minors	*Age of Legal Capacity (Scotland) Act 1991* *Age of Minority Act 1969* (Northern Ireland) *Children (Scotland) Act 1995* *Children Act 1989* *Family Law Reform Act 1969* (England and Wales)
	Consent in special cases	*Children and Young Persons Act 1933*
	Consent—incompetent patient	*Human Rights Act 1998* *Mental Health Act 1983*
6	Confidentiality	*Human Rights Act 1998*
	Disclosure public interest	*Ontario Medicine Act 1991* *Police Act 1964* *Public Interest Disclosure Act 1998*
	data protection	*Access to Health Records Act 1000* (England, Wales, Scotland) *Access to Health Records Act 1994* (Northern Ireland) *Consumer Protection Act 1987* *Data Protection Act 1998*

Continued

Contd.

Chapter	Subject	Related Legislation (UK Unless Stated Otherwise)
	employers/insurers	*Access to Medical Reports Act 1988* (England, Wales, Scotland) *Access to Personal Files and Medical Reports (NI) Order 1991* (Northern Ireland)
	teaching/audit/research	*Data Protection Act 1998*
	adverse drug reactions	*Data Protection Act 1998*
	civil litigation	*Data Protection Act 1998* *Supreme Court Act 1981*
	criminal proceedings	*Criminal Procedure (Scotland) Act 1995* *Criminal Procedure and Investigations Act 1996* *Police and Criminal Evidence Act (PACE) 1984* *Prevention of Terrorism (Temporary Provisions) Act 2000*
	Breach of confidentiality—controlled circumstances	*Abortion Act 1991* *AIDS (Control) Act 1987* *Births and Deaths Registration Act 1953* *Control of Substances Hazardous to Health (COSHH) Regulations* *Factories Act 1895* *Human Fertilisation and Embryology (Disclosure of Information) Act 1992* *Human Fertilisation and Embryology Act 1990* *Misuse of Drugs (Notification and Supply to Addicts) Regulations 1985* *Misuse of Drugs Act 1971* *NHS (Notification of Births and Deaths) Regulations 1982* *NHS (Venereal Disease) Regulations 1974* *Perjury Act 1911* *Prevention of Terrorism (Temporary Provisions) Act 2000* *Public Health (Control of Disease) Act 1984* *Public Health (Infectious Diseases) Regulations 1988* *Road Traffic Act 1988*
7	Risk management	*Health and Safety at Work Act 1974*
	CNST	*NHS and Community Care Act 1990* (Section 21)
8	Health Service Ombudsman	*Health Service Commissioners Act 1993*
9	Contributory negligence	*Social Security Administration Act 1992* (England, Wales, Scotland) *Social Security Administration (Northern Ireland) Act 1992* *Vaccine Damage Payments Act 1979*
	Negligence claim—time limitation	*Limitation Act 1980*
10	General Medical Council: establishment	*Medical Act 1858*
	powers, including discipline	*Medical Act 1983*
	education	*European Specialist Medical Qualifications Order 1995*
	Committee on Professional Performance	*Medical (Professional Performance) Act 1995*
	NMC (UKCC)	*Health Act 1983* *Nurses, Midwives and Health Visitors Act 1979* *Nurses, Midwives and Health Visitors Act 1992* *Nursing and Midwifery Order 2001*
	Professions supplementary to medicine	*Professions Supplementary to Medicine Act 1960*

Chapter	Subject	Related Legislation (UK Unless Stated Otherwise)
	NHS tribunal	*NHS Act 1977* *Tribunals and Inquiries Act 1992*
	Protected disclosure	*Public Interest Disclosure Act 1998*
11	Death certification	*Births and Deaths Registration Act 1953* (England & Wales) *Coroner's Act (Northern Ireland) 1959* *Fatal Accidents and Sudden Deaths Inquiry (Scotland) Act 1976* *Registration of Births, Deaths and Marriages (Scotland) Act 1965*
	Coroner system	*Coroners Act 1988*
	Postmortem/removal of tissue	*Human Tissue Act 1961* *Human Tissue Act 1962* (Northern Ireland)
	Disposal	*Anatomy Act 1984* *Births and Deaths Registration Act 1926*
12	Organ donation, organ retrieval	*Human Tissue Act 1961* *Human Tissue Act 1962* (Northern Ireland)
	Payment for organs	*Human Organ Transplants Act 1989*
	Living donor	*Human Organ Transplants Act 1989* *Human Organ Transplants (Unrelated Persons) Regulations 1989*
13	Physician-assisted suicide	*Burial and Cremation Act 1991* (Holland) *Death with Dignity Act 1994* (USA) *Rights of the Terminally Ill Act 1996* (Northern Territory, Australia) *Termination of Life on Request and Assisted Suicide Review Act 2002* (Holland)
	Advance Directive	*Adults with Incapacity (Scotland) Act 2000* *Children Act 1989* *Mental Health Act 1983* *Natural Death Act of California 1976* (California, USA) *Patient Self-Determination Act 1991* (USA)
14	Infanticide	*Infanticide Act 1938*
	Stillbirth	*Stillbirth (Definition) Act 1992* *Still-Births (Scotland) Act 1938*
	Child destruction	*Infant Life Preservation Act 1929*
	Concealment of birth	*Concealment of Birth (Scotland) Act 1809* *Offences against the Person Act 1861* (England and Wales)
	Children Acts	*Children Act 1989* (England and Wales) *Children (Scotland) Act 1995*
15	Mental health	*Mental Health Act 1983* *Mental Health Act 1984* (Scotland)
16	Drink driving	*Road Traffic Act 1988*
17	Drugs prescribing	*Medicinal Products: Prescription by Nurses Act 1992*
	misuse	*Dangerous Drugs Acts 1965, 1967* *Drugs (Prevention of Misuse) Act 1964* *Misuse of Drugs (Notification and Supply to Addicts) Regulations 1973* *Misuse of Drugs (Safe Custody) Regulations 1973* *Misuse of Drugs Act 1971* (England, Wales, Scotland) *Misuse of Drugs Regulations 1985*
	Safety of medicines	*Medicines Act 1968*

CNST, Clinical Negligence Scheme for Trusts; *NMC*, Nursing and Midwifery Council; *UKCC*, United Kingdom Central Council for Nursing, Midwifery and Health Visiting.

Glossary

Absolute privilege complete immunity from an action for libel or slander even if what was said was motivated by malice

Actual bodily harm (ABH) intentional assault occasioning physical injury

Actus Reus the act of commission of a criminal offence

Admiralty law applies to British and foreign vessels and involves mostly civil matters

Advance Decision a statement made by a mentally competent adult that gives instructions about how he would wish to be treated in the event of any future loss of mental capacity

Alternative dispute resolution an alternative to civil litigation, where a third party acts as a mediator but his decision is not binding and the disputing parties must negotiate their own settlement

Arbitration an adjudication process that operates outside court, where a third party reviews the case and makes a decision that is binding on both parties

Balance of probabilities the account most likely to be the true version of events

Battery infliction of personal violence

'Best interests' decisions choices made on the behalf of incompetent patients to provide the most beneficial treatment

Body packers ('mules') people who transport drugs in various body cavities

Body stuffers ('swallowers') people who swallow drugs when arrested

Bolam standard a healthcare professional must act in accordance with a responsible and competent body of relevant professional opinion if he is not to be found negligent

Brain stem death the point at which mechanical life support should be discontinued

Caldicott guardian a member of staff (usually the medical director) appointed by each NHS Trust to oversee issues of confidentiality

Causation the link between actionable harm and the breach of duty of care

Child destruction the killing of a fetus in utero after 28 weeks

Civil law a private matter; proceedings are usually instituted by the injured party

Common assault threatening behaviour

Common law case or judge-made law

Concealment of birth the hiding of a body to conceal the fact of birth

Consent (implied, express) (i) *implied*—behavioural, e.g. a patient voluntarily undresses for examination; (ii) *express*—the patient gives permission orally or in writing

Contributory negligence actions of a claimant that makes or made the alleged injury worse

Criminal law relates to a crime that directly and seriously threatens the well-being of the general population

Date of knowledge date on which alleged negligence occurred or when the patient became aware of the effects

Death (definition of) irreversible loss of the capacity for consciousness, combined with irreversible loss of the capacity to breathe

Death certificate (stillbirth, neonatal, cause of death) (i) *stillbirth*—after 24 weeks' gestation; (ii) *neonatal*—any death up to 28 days of age; (iii) *Medical Certificate of Cause of Death*—all other deaths

Dependence syndrome compulsion to use drugs with an over-riding focus on drug-seeking behaviour + ≥ 1 of the following:
1. Tolerance—the amount of drug needed to give the desired effect rises
2. Withdrawal—both physical & psychological symptoms on stopping use
3. Use of drug to relieve or avoid withdrawal symptoms

Discovery the point where all parties must produce all documents in their possession relevant to an issue in litigation

Dismissal (with notice, action short of dismissal, summary dismissal, constructive) (i) *dismissal with notice* is used for serious offences where the safety of patients is not at risk; (ii) *action short of dismissal* is used for less serious offences and includes transfer to other work or to a different location or up to 4 weeks of unpaid leave; (iii) *summary* *dismissal* is immediate dismissal without notice and is used for very serious offences where the welfare of the patients has been put in jeopardy; (iv) *constructive dismissal* is behaviour of an employer such that the employee is entitled to terminate his employment and consider himself dismissed

Doctrine of necessity medical treatment of an unconscious patient in the absence of consent in the 'best interests' of the patient

Doctrine of 'double-effect' the healthcare professional can foresee that the consequences of his actions are likely to be beneficial to the patient but could also be detrimental

Ecclesiastical law concerned with regulation of church affairs

Euthanasia active intervention to end life

Evidence (direct, circumstantial, hearsay) (i) *direct evidence* requires no mental processing by the judge or jury; (ii) *circumstantial evidence* requires the judge or jury to draw inferences; (iii) *hearsay evidence* is reported speech

Examination-in-chief the first line of questioning faced by a witness in court

Frozen awareness either incapable or fearful of displaying any emotion

'Gardening leave' leave on full pay for a period not usually exceeding 6 months to allow recovery from illness

Gillick competent a minor of any age considered to have sufficient understanding and intelligence to give or refuse consent

Grievous bodily harm (GBH) intentional wounding resulting in a breach in the skin

Industrial law relates to conditions of employment, trade unions and industrial relations

Infanticide the deliberate killing of an infant under the age of 12 months

Intimate body search physical examination of the orifices (ears, nostrils, mouth, rectum and vagina)

Intoximeter a machine used to measure the concentration of alcohol in a breath sample

Letter of administration allows the personal representatives of a person who died intestate to give consent of the behalf of the deceased

Letter of Claim gives the dates of alleged negligent treatment and the events giving rise to the claim

Letter of Response reply to Letter of Claim, commenting on the events if they are disputed, with details of any other documentation upon which the defendant intends to rely

Living Will See Advance Decision

Medicinal purpose relates to drugs used in the diagnosis, treatment or prevention of disease, induction of anaesthesia, contraception or any other permanent or temporary effect on physiological function

Medicines (POMs, P, GSL, unlicensed) (i) *prescription-only medicines (POMs)* are those that may only be supplied or administered on the instruction of a doctor, dentist or paramedic-prescriber; (ii) *pharmacy-only medicines (P)* are those that may only be bought from a registered pharmacy, under the supervision of a pharmacist; (iii) *general sale list medicines (GSLs)* are those that can be bought from any retail outlet; (iv) *unlicensed medicines* are those with no product licence and no manufacturer liability

Mens rea the intention to commit a criminal offence

Mental disorder mental illness, arrested or incomplete development of mind, psychopathic disorder or any other disorder or disability of mind

Mental impairment a state of arrested or incomplete development of mind which includes significant impairment of intelligence and social functioning and is associated with abnormally aggressive or seriously irresponsible conduct on the part of the person concerned

Newton hearing occurs when the accused pleads guilty and the judge elects to hear from the prosecution and defence in order to decide sentencing

Orders of court—children (contact, prohibited steps, residence, specific issues) (i) *contact order* defines persons with whom the child must be allowed to have contact; (ii) *prohibited steps order* stops a person with parental responsibility from making certain decisions over the child's welfare without recourse to the courts; (iii) *residence order* defines where and with whom the child will live; (iv) *specific issues order* gives directions for dealing with a particular aspect of the child's care

Patient group directions (PGD) the supply and administration of a named medicine or vaccine in a known clinical situation where patients may not be identified prior to arrival

Permanent vegetative state (PVS) the brain stem still functions but cortex does not, so the patient can breathe unaided and the autonomic nervous system works but he cannot see, hear, speak, feel pain or move voluntarily

Personal misconduct inappropriate behaviour unrelated to clinical skills

Physician-assisted suicide a doctor prescribes a lethal drug but it is either administered by the patient or by a third party

Polymerase chain reaction (PCR) new, more accurate method of DNA profiling using minute quantities of material; chance of a random match <1 in several millions

Professional incompetence inadequate or poor performance of clinical skills or judgement

Professional misconduct inappropriate behaviour arising during the exercise of clinical skills

'Proofing' the defendant's solicitors prepare answers to the particulars of the claim

Protected disclosure disclosure of confidential information concerning matters of public interest to only the relevant bodies

Psychopathic disorder a persistent disorder or disability of mind (whether or not including significant impairment of intelligence) that results in abnormally aggressive or seriously irresponsible conduct on the part of the person concerned

Quantifiable harm disability, loss or injury suffered as a result of negligence by another

Quantum the amount of financial compensation for the harm suffered as a result of negligence by another

Risk management the ability to detect, analyse and learn from adverse events

Service law applies to all serving members of the Navy, Air Force and Army; administered through courts martial

Severe mental impairment a state of arrested or incomplete development of mind which includes severe impairment of intelligence and social functioning; it is associated with abnormally aggressive or seriously irresponsible conduct on the part of the person concerned

Shaken baby syndrome a clinical and pathological entity characterised by retinal and subdural and/ or subarachnoid haemorrhages with minimal or absent signs of external trauma

Statute law law that is enacted by the Parliament

Subpoena a writ calling a person to attend at court

'Substitutive judgement' decisions the decision-maker must provide the treatment that the patient would have chosen if he had still competent; tend to be based on quality, rather than quantity of life

Tin ear bruising of the pinna of the ear caused by slap to the side of the head

Tolerance physiological changes within the body so that larger amounts of alcohol or drugs of addiction must be consumed in order to achieve the same effects

Tort a civil wrong, dealt with through civil proceedings

Tutor-dative a person appointed under the *Adults with Incapacity (Scotland) Act 2000* who has the authority to make medical decisions on behalf of an incompetent patient

Vicarious liability legal responsibility for the actions of juniors or other staff

Withdrawal (from drug dependence) both physical and psychological symptoms if the drug is not taken

Withdrawal/withholding of treatment treatment is either stopped or not started on the basis that it would be of no benefit to the patient

Witness (of fact, professional, expert) (i) *witness of fact* is one who gives factual evidence; (ii) a *professional witness* is one who also provides factual evidence but can give some opinions; (iii) an *expert witness* is one who provides both fact and opinion evidence and guides the court over matters that are the subject of special expertise

Xenotransplantation the transfer of viable cells, tissues or organs between species

Yellow Card scheme method by which healthcare professionals can report any adverse drug reactions to the Committee on Safety of Medicines

Index

Note: Page numbers followed by '*f*' indicate figures, '*t*' indicate tables and '*b*' indicate boxes. *NI*, Northern Ireland.